Intravenous therapy
A HANDBOOK FOR PRACTICE

Intravenous therapy
A HANDBOOK FOR PRACTICE

CHARLENE DIANNE COCO, R.N., B.S.N.

Instructor, Louisiana State University Medical Center
School of Nursing, Associate Degree Program,
New Orleans, Louisiana

with 56 *illustrations*

The C. V. Mosby Company

ST. LOUIS • TORONTO • LONDON   1980

The C. V. Mosby Company
11830 Westline Industrial Drive, St. Louis, Missouri 63141

Library of Congress Cataloging in Publication Data

Coco, Charlene Dianne, 1943-
  Intravenous therapy.

  Bibliography: p.
  Includes index.
    1. Intravenous therapy—Handbooks, manuals, etc.
I. Title. [DNLM: 1. Infusions, Parenteral.
WB354 C667i]
RM170.C62   615'.63   79-19930
ISBN 0-8016-0995-X

GW/VH/VH 9 8 7 6 5 4 3 2 1   05/C/603

*To my colleagues in practice
and to Papa,
for without these people
this work would not have been accomplished*

Preface

In the United States approximately 10 million patients receive some form of intravenous therapy each year.

In a typical acute care setting one can expect at least 25% of all patients admitted to receive either continuous or intermittent intravenous therapy.

Intravenous therapy has increased drastically over the last 15 years largely because of advances in oncologic pharmacotherapeutics and parenteral hyperalimentation. Other therapies include restoration of lost or depleted body fluid and electrolytes, replacement of blood, provision of nutrition, administration of medications, and maintenance of venous lines, which can be useful during periods of crisis.

The equipment, policies, and procedures regarding intravenous therapy vary widely from hospital to hospital. Specific infection control techniques are required in order to protect the patient from nosocomial infections.

The nurse is the primary deliverer of intravenous therapy and, as such, must adhere to specific legal guidelines.

The major objectives of this work are to:

Increase the nurse's knowledge of the rationale underlying intravenous therapy and venipuncture

Assist the nurse in learning to use this knowledge clinically in order to recognize both therapeutic and deleterious effects of intravenous therapy and venipuncture

Assist the nurse in learning to identify appropriate nursing actions relating to intravenous therapy and venipuncture

Present the legal aspects of intravenous therapy and venipuncture

Assist the nurse in learning the pharmacodynamics of intravenous therapy*

---

*From Delbueno, D., et al.: Teaching pharmacology, Nurs. Outlook **19:**6, June 1971. Copyright 1971 by the American Journal of Nursing Co.

The focus of this work is on intravenous therapy as it relates to the adult patient. Specific information on the disease entities and drugs mentioned can be found in other texts. The list of references should serve as at least an initial source for searching the literature.

Charlene Coco

Acknowledgments

The following persons and institutions have been instrumental in making this work become a reality:

Alton Ochsner Medical Foundation, Hospital Division, Departments of Nursing, Pharmacy, Blood Bank, IV Team, Emergency Room, and Public Relations, New Orleans, Louisiana

Bohm, J., R.N., Head Nurse, IV Team, Hotel Dieu Hospital, New Orleans, Louisiana

Bouvette, J., R.N., Neurosurgical Nurse Clinician, Alton Ochsner Medical Foundation, Hospital Division, Department of Nursing Service, New Orleans, Louisiana

Boyce, R., Photographer, Alton Ochsner Medical Foundation, New Orleans, Louisiana

Buisson, C., R.N., Ph.D., Continuing Education Coordinator, Louisiana State University School of Nursing, New Orleans, Louisiana

Capaci, T., R.N., Assistant Head Nurse, IV Team, Hotel Dieu Hospital, New Orleans, Louisiana

Coco, H., Ph.D., Clinical Psychologist, Ponchartrain Mental Health Center, New Orleans, Louisiana

Gentry, J., R.N., Associate Hospital Director/Director of Nursing Service, Alton Ochsner Medical Foundation, Hospital Division, New Orleans, Louisiana

Gros, C., B.S., Chief, Respiratory Therapy Department, Humana, Inc., Marksville General Hospital, Marksville, Louisiana

Hart, P., R.N., M.N., Assistant Professor of Nursing, Louisiana State University at Alexandria, Alexandria, Louisiana

Johnson, P., M.D., Department of Emergency Medicine, Alton Ochsner Medical Foundation, New Orleans, Louisiana

Liles, S., R.N., B.S.N.Ed., Education and Training Specialist, Alton Ochsner Medical Foundation, New Orleans, Louisiana

Louisiana State Nurses' Association Continuing Education Project and Louisiana State University School of Nursing, New Orleans, Louisiana

Mearns, G., B.A., Journalist, New Orleans, Louisiana

Melancon, T., J.D., Marksville, Louisiana

Monti, J., R.N., B.S.N., Associate Director of Nursing, Alton Ochsner Medical Foundation, Hospital Division, New Orleans, Louisiana

Neel, J., B.S.N., Instructor in Nursing, Louisiana State University at Alexandria, Alexandria, Louisiana

Odom, B., R. N., M.Ed., Director, Division of Nursing, Louisiana State University at Alexandria, Alexandria, Louisiana

Pickard, E., Typist, Marksville, Louisiana

Primm, M., R.N., M.S.N., Executive Director, Louisiana State Nurses' Association, New Orleans, Louisiana

Risey, B., R.N., M.Ed., Assistant Professor of Nursing, Louisiana State University at New Orleans, New Orleans, Louisiana

Sibille, L., R.N., B.S.N., Intravenous Staff Developer, Children's Hospital, New Orleans, Louisiana

Contents

Chapter 1

Factors affecting practice

The registered nurse is the primary deliverer of intravenous therapy. Few courses specific to intravenous therapy are available in schools of nursing. Most schools integrate intravenous therapy training in courses related to surgical nursing, while some schools do not include intravenous therapy in their curricula. As a result, nurses in practice possess varying degrees of knowledge and skill.

Evaluation of the competency of each nurse charged with the responsibility of delivering intravenous therapy is a method of assuring quality care. This can be accomplished through written, oral, and practical examinations.

Areas of competency include an understanding of the functions of the cardiovascular system; fluid, electrolyte, and acid-base balance; pharmacodynamics; and the nurse's ability to use equipment and recognize patient responses.

When necessary, nurses should complete a prescribed course of study related to the theoretical and practical aspects of intravenous therapy. Successful completion of the course is ascertained when the nurse achieves a satisfactory score on written, oral, and practical examinations.

Once competency is realized, specific guidelines for practice should be established and adhered to. These guidelines, or statements of general policy, should comply with each state's nurse practice act, individual hospital policy, and procedure and common practice in each geographical area.

LAWS GOVERNING THE PRACTICE OF NURSING

State nurse practice acts and state boards of nursing govern the practice of nursing. Changes and amendments to laws relating to nursing practice are carried out through the state's legislative system.

State nurse practice acts vary, and as such, the nurse should follow that written in one's own state.

The Louisiana State Nurse Practice Act (1976), as an example of the law, states:

> . . . said practice shall include the supervision and instruction of professional and non-professional personnel associated with nursing functions and may include the performance of such additional acts as are recognized by the nursing profession as proper to the practice of nursing and which are authorized by the board.
>
> Selected nursing functions may be delegated to licensed or unlicensed personnel, unless objected to by the attending physician or dentist and/or the medical staff of the institution.
>
> Delegation of such functions may not necessarily require the personal presence of the delegating registered nurse at the place where such functions are performed, unless such personal presence is necessary to provide patient care of the same quality as provided by the registered nurse.

The Louisiana State Nurses' Association (LSNA, 1977) stated:

> . . . the purpose of the Nurse Practice Act is to protect the public. The Board of Nursing is delegated administrative and implementation functions and is charged with guarding the public welfare. It is therefore proper for the Board of Nursing to issue interpretations and rules and regulations concerning nursing functions performed by nurses or those whom nurses supervise.

LSNA (1977) further stated:

> . . . a licensed practical nurse employed by a hospital must be supervised by a registered nurse. Physicians on the staff of a hospital are not employees and therefore cannot be responsible for the activities of hospital employees. It would be the professional nurse who would be liable for acts of the licensed practical nurse, not the physician.
>
> The medical staff does not establish the policies and procedures for the performance and functions of nurses employed by a hospital. This is done by the nursing service director and hospital administrator in consultation with the professional nursing staff. The staff physicians do not evaluate the competence of nurses employed by the hospital. This evaluation originates with the immediate supervisor of the individual nurse.
>
> The board of directors of a hospital is, of course, ultimately responsible for the performance of all employees. However, members of hospital boards of directors are primarily persons not engaged in the practice of medicine or nursing. They are not, therefore, qualified by experience or education to evaluate technical or professional competence.
>
> The action of professional nurses must be based on individual nurses' understanding of cause and effect. The administration of intravenous fluids or medications is a serious matter. Drugs have an immediate action when injected directly into the circulatory system. The course of study of a practical nurse is not of sufficient depth to provide the knowl-

edge needed to understand the action of drugs administered by this route. A professional nurse would be derelict in her responsibility for the safety of a patient if she allowed a licensed practical to administer drugs intravenously.

The technique of puncturing a vein is not complex. However, the observation of a patient to determine the effect of the drug administered requires substantial specialized knowledge and skill.

When duties other than the most basic are delegated to the licensed practical nurse or to nonlicensed personnel, it is advisable that specialized training in the area and documentation of successful completion of a prescribed course be provided. This would include passing a test based on the course objectives.

Some basic duties related to intravenous therapy are calculating and regulating flow rates, choosing the fluid according to the physician's order, admixing routine and continuous infusions, observing the IV site for infiltration of the fluid into the surrounding tissues, and recording of information such as the type of solution, amount, medication added, and flow rate.

It appears that the quality of care of the patient is diluted when intravenous therapy is delegated to licensed and unlicensed personnel, since the depth of knowledge required in understanding the circulatory system, its compartments, and fluid and electrolyte balance is inadequate. There is far more involved than the mere technical aspects.

Primm (1978) stated:

> L.S.N.A. recognizes the dilemma which confronts the profession, the Board of Nursing and the public. In hospitals and nursing homes . . . patients are receiving intravenous fluids and medications which are administered by licensed practical nurses. We know the ideal is not always possible, but as professional nurses, we cannot approve of the performance of dangerous procedures by inadequately prepared persons.
>
> L.S.N.A. believes that the person performing the nursing function of administering intravenous fluids and medications must have a sound background in pharmacology. This background must be based on knowledge of biochemistry and physiology. This preparation cannot be obtained through a short course or on the job training.
>
> If it can be demonstrated that licensed practical nurses, or any health worker functioning under the supervision of the registered nurses, have the preparation to perform this procedure safely, then there is no problem. The welfare of the public will not be in jeopardy.
>
> Until the public can be assured that nursing personnel other than registered nurses can administer intravenous fluids and medications safely, L.S.N.A. believes this must continue to be a function of the registered nurse.
>
> The setting of rules and regulations may make this a legal function but not necessarily a safe procedure. If the need for nursing personnel

other than registered nurses to administer intravenous fluids and medications can be established, more than rules and regulations are needed. This would have implications for change in the educational programs of those involved.

L.S.N.A. recognizes that emergency medical technicians do administer intravenous medications at sites of emergencies. However, these technicians function under the supervision of physicians, not nurses. It is therefore incumbent upon physicians to assure the public that these technicians are practicing safely.*

In essence the nurse has a right and responsibility to refuse to perform a function should she or he feel unqualified or that the function is not safe practice. In addition, the nurse has the right and responsibility to seek training in order that her or his level of knowledge remains in keeping with what is required to perform daily duties.

Following are excerpts regarding the legal responsibilities of the nurse as collected by Gentry (1975):

> The nurse maintains individual competence in nursing practice, recognizing and accepting responsibility for individual actions and judgments (both dependent and independent nursing functions). (ANA Code for Professional Nurses)
>
> The nurse will not take or knowingly administer any harmful drug. (Nightingale Pledge)
>
> No person may absolve another of liability. No physician may order a nurse to perform an act and assure her that he will assume full responsibility. The nurse who acts pursuant to such an understanding without an appreciation of the cause and effect of the order she is to execute, renders herself and the patient a disservice. The law is clear that a nurse is required to understand the procedure or technique she is directed to apply. (Lesnik and Anderson, 1962)
>
> The nurse's right to perform any function involving a medical act is conditioned absolutely upon her capacity of understanding to execute the same. Clearly, the nurse is entitled to no consideration in a malpractice case because she alleges that she was ordered to perform that function. No order may contravene the inherent obligation to secure the patient's safety. (Lesnik and Anderson, 1962)

HOSPITAL POLICY

Webster's Dictionary (1963) defines a policy as "a projected program consisting of desired objectives and the means to achieve them." The *American Heritage Dictionary* (1973) states that "policies should be designed in a manner in which decisions are influenced and determined."

A policy related to intravenous therapy should spell out who is to

---

*From Primm, M.: L.S.N.A. gives views on IV therapy to Board of Nursing, Pelican News **34:**1, Spring, 1978.

perform the therapy, what can be administered, age of patient restrictions, when the therapy is to be performed (that is, in some areas intravenous teams provide all services for 12 to 16 hours a day, after which the general nursing staff is responsible), responsibilities of the physician, and responsibilities of the nurse. Only that which is written, approved, and accepted should be performed.

The boxed material is a sample policy taken in part from the Alton Ochsner Medical Foundation, Hospital Division, Department of Nursing Service, New Orleans.

POLICY
Intravenous medications and venipuncture by registered nurses

Registered nurses trained in intravenous techniques may start infusions and transfusions. The nurse may also add blood to an in-progress infusion provided the infusion is first flushed with normal saline. She may also administer intravenous medications via the push method and by venipuncture provided the drug ordered is on the approved list.

The policy regarding venipuncture applies to patients 4 years of age and older.

All nurses trained in intravenous techniques must have documentation of their ability. This documentation is to be carried out by the assigned registered nurse from the staff development department. Documentation follows successful completion of the hospital's prescribed 20-hour course on intravenous techniques.

Hours

Infusions, transfusions, and adding blood: after 9:30 PM on weekdays and after 4:30 PM on weekends and holidays (when no intravenous team nurse is available).

IV push medications and administration of medications by venipuncture whenever ordered by the physician and only when drug ordered is on approved list.

Responsibility of physicians

Infusions, transfusions, and medications to be given by the intravenous route must be ordered by the physician with the following information included: (1) rate of speed for infusions and transfusions or the length of time necessary for administration and (2) dosage of medication, route, and type of needle to be used as indicated. Method of IV administration must be specified, that is, IV by continuous flow, piggyback, or push.

Blood specimens for type and cross matching and type and holds are to be collected by the physician after 4:30 PM except in certain specialty areas where policies vary.

Continued.

POLICY—cont'd
Responsibility of nurses

Successful completion of prescribed course in intravenous techniques.

Thorough knowledge of drugs on approved list, including cause and effect.

Ability to differentiate between drugs that can and cannot be administered with special monitoring and those that must be administered only in the presence of a physician.

The registered nurse is not permitted to start infusions containing levarterenol bitartrate or metaraminol bitartrate.

The nurse may start an infusion using a No. 19-, 20-, 21-, 22-, 23-, or 25-gauge scalp vein needle.

The nurse may also start infusions using a No. 16-, 18-, or 20-gauge over-the-needle type cannula when ordered by the physician or when preoperative infusions are started.

IV push medications and medications administered by venipuncture are to be administered using No. 23-, 22-, or 21-gauge needles.

Should an infusion need flushing prior to injecting a medication, as in the case of incompatibilities with drugs and in-progress infusions, the nurse is to follow specific procedure as to the amount and type of solution to use before and after injecting the medication. This extra solution is to be included in the patient's intake record.

If no vein is available, or in doubtful situations, venipuncture becomes the responsibility of the physician.

Insertion of intravenous catheters of the in-the-needle type that exceed 3.5 inches in length is considered beyond the scope of nursing practice. Cutdowns and insertion of subclavian catheters are to be done by the physician.

Drug lists

Each drug administered to a patient via the vascular system is potentially lethal. It is advisable to have a list of drugs approved for administration by the IV push route.

The list serves several purposes including protection for the physician, nurse, and patient.

All drugs on the list should be reviewed and approved as safe when administered as recommended. This narrows the margin for error, since drugs not recommended for intravenous use would be excluded from the list.

Drug lists may be prepared whereby there is a delineation of drugs that can be administered by nurses in general care areas and intensive care areas. Special monitoring and the presence of a physician will be necessary during the administration of certain drugs.

Listing of drugs allows the nurse to become aware of drugs she or he will be expected to administer. This affords the nurse the opportunity to become expert regarding drug actions, indications and uses, dosages, dilutions and rates of administration, side effects, and antidotes.

The agency's pharmacy and therapeutics committee (P and T committee) should be responsible for preparing the drug list. Additions and deletions to the list should also be its responsibility.

P and T committees are composed of physicians, pharmacists, and nurses. This balance of three important disciplines assures that prior to acceptance or rejection of drugs for intravenous push administration, factors involving chemistry, pharmacology, pathophysiology, clinical efficacy, and patient response will be considered.

The P and T committee member has the opportunity to serve the important functions of educating the staff in the proper selection and use of drugs, monitoring the use of drugs, and collecting, evaluating, and reporting data pertinent to the adverse effects of drugs.

Listing of drugs administered by way of continuous infusion and piggyback may be impractical since the numbers are so great.

Following is an example of a list of drugs approved for IV push administration*:

1. Drugs to be administered by registered nurses in general and intensive care areas:
   Acetazolamide sodium (Diamox)
   Amethopterin (Methotrexate)
   Azathioprine sodium (Imuran)
   Chlordiazepoxide hydrochloride (Librium)
   Colchicine
   Cyclophosphamide (Cytoxan)
   Cytarabine (Cytosar)
   Dexamethasone sodium phosphate (Decadron)
   Dextrose (glucose 50%)
   Diazepam (Valium)
   Diphenhydramine hydrochloride (Benadryl)
   Ethacrynic acid (Edecrin)
   Fluorouracil (5-Fluorouracil)

---

*Taken in part from Approved Drug List, Alton Ochsner Medical Foundation, Hospital Division, Department of Nursing Service, New Orleans, Louisiana, 1977.

Folinic acid (Leucovorin Calcium)
Furosemide (Lasix)
Heparin sodium (Lipo-Hepin)
Hydralazine hydrochloride (Apresoline)
Hydrocortisone phosphate
Hydrocortisone sodium succinate (Solu-Cortef)
Hydromorphone hydrochloride (Dilaudid)
Menadiol sodium diphosphate (Synkayvite)
Menadione sodium bisulfite (Hykinone)
Meperidine hydrochloride (Demerol)
Methyldopate hydrochloride (Aldomet)
Methylprednisolone sodium succinate (Solu-Medrol)
Morphine sulfate
Naloxone hydrochloride (Narcan)
Phenytoin sodium (Dilantin)
Phytonadione (Aquamephyton)
Propantheline bromide (Pro-Banthine)
Sodium bicarbonate

2. Drugs to be administered by registered nurses in intensive care areas (recovery room, intensive care, coronary care, emergency room, nursery, delivery, operating room, dialysis):

Alphaprodine hydrochloride (Nisentil)
Amobarbital sodium (Amytal Sodium)
Atropine
Caffeine sodium benzoate
Calcium chloride
Calcium gluconate
Chlorpromazine hydrochloride (Thorazine)
Deslanoside (Cedilanid-D)
Digitoxin
Digoxin (Lanoxin)
Doxapram hydrochloride (Dopram)
Edrophonium chloride (Tensilon)
Ephedrine
Epinephrine hydrochloride (Adrenalin Chloride)
Glucagon
Glycopyrrolate (Robinul)
Innovar
Insulin, regular
Isoproterenol hydrochloride (Isuprel)
Levallorphan tartrate (Lorfan)
Lidocaine hydrochloride (Xylocaine)

Magnesium sulfate
Methoxamine hydrochloride (Vasoxyl)
Methylergonovine maleate (Methergine)
Nalorphine hydrochloride (Nalline)
Neostigmine methylsulfate (Prostigmin)
Oxytocin (Pitocin)
Pancuronium bromide (Pavulon)
Phenobarbital sodium (Luminal)
Phentolamine mesylate (Regitine)
Phenylephrine hydrochloride (Neo-Synephrine)
Procainamide hydrochloride (Pronestyl)
Promethazine hydrochloride (Phenergan)
Propranolol hydrochloride (Inderal)
Protamine sulfate
Secobarbital sodium (Seconal)
Succinylcholine chloride (Anectine)
Tubocurarine chloride (curare)

Should a physician or group of physicians order drugs not on the list, it is recommended that the nursing staff or physician(s) present the drug to the P and T committee for review.

It is advisable to stay within the limits that have been set. Should any policy become obsolete because of changes in practice, or should a policy be considered unrealistic by the medical or nursing staff, a proposal for change should be presented to the agency's policy and procedure committee. The appropriate lines of authority should be followed in order to effect this process.

PROCEDURES

The *American Heritage Dictionary* (1973) defines a procedure as "a set of established forms for conducting business or public affairs; a series of steps or course of action." *Webster's Dictionary* (1968) defines a procedure as "a particular course of action or a series of steps followed in a regular, orderly, and defined way."

Included among the procedures related to intravenous therapy are intravenous infusion, intravenous push administration of drugs, intravenous piggyback administration of drugs, parenteral hyperalimentation, intralipid therapy, and blood administration. Details for these procedures can be found in subsequent chapters.

Each procedure must be performed as written, but modifications are sometimes necessary. All modifications are based on the individual patient and his or her condition.

Should a procedure become obsolete because of changes in practice, or should it be considered unrealistic, proposals for change should be presented to the agency's policy and procedures committee.

NURSES' BODY OF KNOWLEDGE AND LEVEL OF EXPERTISE

In order to safely and effectively perform a function, a nurse must be educated and demonstrate mastery of the specific function.

It is necessary that in-service training be provided to all nurses who lack in-depth knowledge and skill in intravenous techniques.

In-service training, which may be 20 to 40 hours in length, is composed of teaching-learning activities related to hospital policy; legalities; infection control; anatomy and physiology of the cardiovascular system, fluid, electrolyte, and acid-base balance; preparation and administration of intravenous medications; techniques of venipuncture; patient preparation; hazards and complications; blood therapy; and return demonstration of all related procedures.

In order that the nurse gain experience in venipuncture and starting infusions, practical training should be provided. This training should be provided by IV team members or by a nurse who has been approved to perform this function.

Continuous learning and updating of knowledge and skill is necessary to maintain excellence.

Creighton (1970) stated:

> It appears that the nurse is confronted with a paradox. Either she limits her knowledge and outlook because 'nurses do not need to know that' or she expands her knowledge and horizons and increases her frustrations in the practice of her profession. Irrespective of the extent to which the nurse might desire to limit her own professional development, there is little basis in fact for the statement that the nurse does not need to know many things. True she does not need to know certain fields to the same depth as the physician because she is not usually involved in differential diagnosis. However, there is no way for her to safely practice nursing while at the same time limiting her own knowledge. She has to constantly read and inform herself of current acceptable and/or recommended practices simply out of self-preservation, to protect herself from legal action. One cannot claim freedom from liability for failure to use due care on the basis that others are performing in the same negligent or careless manner.*

It is the wise nurse who stays within the limits that have been set by the employing agency and the nurse practice act. It is also the wise nurse who continuously updates her or his knowledge and skill.

---

*From Creighton, H.: Changing legal attitudes: the effect of the law on nursing, New York, 1974, National League for Nursing, p. 2.

REPORTING AND RECORDING

Reporting and recording of the administered therapy and the patient's response is of major importance. Documentation of care and the patient's responses to care is part of the nursing process.

All unusual occurrences should be immediately reported to the attending physician, since this may necessitate emergency measures or alterations in the therapeutic plan.

Discrepancies related to the physician's order should be called to the physician's attention. Examples of this are unclear handwriting, missing components such as drug strength and dosage, and indeterminable routes of administration. The IV route of administration would need clarification, since IV can mean continuous, push, or piggyback.

MALPRACTICE INSURANCE

Today is an age of the lawsuit-conscious consumer. Following are points to remember when dealing with potential malpractice-oriented patients:

From the viewpoint of malpractice claims prevention nothing is more effective than giving the highest quality nursing care in accordance with recognized practices and procedures.

Psychological factors play an extremely important role as determinants of malpractice suits. More often than not a patient's decision to sue, although triggered by some adverse medical event, is one way the patient can obtain revenge for what he considers unsatisfactory treatment (in the psychological sense) on the part of the nurse.

Since malpractice claims are founded in part upon the daily interaction between nurse and patient, the nurse's personality plays a significant role in fostering or prevention of malpractice claims.

Because the psychological component can greatly influence a patient to sue or not to sue a nurse, all nurses should become familiar with the principles of patient psychology.

Understanding patient attitudes and behavior will not only prevent malpractice suits but will stimulate the patient's participation in his treatment.

By definition, patient-centered treatment focuses on the patient rather than the task, and this personal approach is calculated to be more beneficial to patient and nurse alike.

Patients should be encouraged to participate in their care to the greatest extent practicable, thereby a more wholesome therapeutic relationship between patient and nurse being assured.

The nurse should consciously try to develop effective interpersonal relationships with her patients and should demonstrate by her words and actions that she not only cares for but cares about her patients.*

---

*From Gentry, J.: Excerpts from a collection of papers on the legal responsibilities of the nurse, New Orleans, 1973, Alton Ochsner Medical Foundation, Hospital Division, Department of Nursing Service.

Most agencies have some type of liability or malpractice insurance for their employees. It is advisable to be informed as to exactly what coverage is provided. Some nurses own a personal insurance policy in order to supplement what is provided by the agency.

LOOSE TALK SYNDROME

The loose talk syndrome is a condition that affects some members of the health care team. It implies that patients are unintentionally informed of unusual occurrences in their care. The patient may be informed through verbal or nonverbal means. For example, nurse to patient: "My, your IV is infiltrated. How long has it been this way? It should have been removed hours ago!" Patient to attorney: "The nurse told me it was wrong so I sued." The patient won.

INFORMED CONSENT

Informed consent is a form of protection for the patient, the agency, and the agency's representatives.

Clearly explain all therapies to the patient. With an understanding of what is to happen and the possible dangers, the patient has a right to consent to or refuse the therapy.

ERRORS

All errors pose a serious threat to the patient. Errors can be classified as minor and major. Minor errors cause little or no harm to the patient, while major errors are life-threatening.

Errors are usually committed out of failure in basic steps of policies, procedures, and medication administration. Distractions are also a causative factor.

It is essential that nurses read labels on medication containers three times, follow the five rights of medication administration, and document all phases of the therapy.

Should an error occur, avoid panic. Steps to resuscitate the patient should be taken as necessary. Notify the physician and prepare an antidote in case one is needed. Discontinue the pernicious drug, fluid, or blood.

Evaluation of the reasons why the error was committed should serve the purpose of preventing future occurrences.

INCIDENT REPORTS

The incident report serves as a detailed account of accidents and unusual occurrences. Once completed, the report is reviewed by selected members of nursing and agency administration, agency attorney, and insurance consultant. It is later filed pending further review.

Prepare the report in duplicate and include the patient's name, room number, age, diagnosis, and a detailed description of the accident or unusual occurrence. Include, in addition, vital signs, patient's response, x-rays, diagnostic tests, and treatments utilized to restore the patient to his or her original state, names of witnesses, and the name of the physician notified.

Document the incident, patient's response and treatment, and physician notified in the nurses' notes. The word "error" and the fact that the incident report was prepared is usually omitted from the nurses' notes.

ADVERSE REACTIONS

Report and record any adverse effects the patient may have from intravenous therapy. Include all signs, symptoms, treatment, and outcome. Inform the physician in detail of adverse effects. Encourage the physician to examine the patient and to draw a diagram on the chart indicating such things as the location or site of phlebitis and areas of pain and infiltration.

BLOOD ADMINISTRATION

In most states blood therapy is considered a service rather than a product. As such, blood is not subject to the Pure Food and Drug Act. Agencies are therefore not considered responsible should a patient develop hepatitis or other complications, providing that a consent form is signed by the patient.

Nurses and agencies are considered responsible for checking blood prior to administration, since it is supplied by the agency and the nurse is an employee representing the agency.

It is advisable within the blood administration policy that two parties, registered nurses or physicians, are to check blood prior to its administration.

Following the check, all discrepancies regarding blood should be reported to the blood bank representative. These discrepancies must be corrected by the blood bank representative prior to blood administration.

INVESTIGATIONAL AND EXPERIMENTAL DRUGS

It is preferred that the ordering physician administer investigational and experimental drugs.

When these drugs are approved by the P and T committee, when cause and effect is known, and when there is a consent form signed by the patient, it is acceptable for nurses to administer investigational and experimental drugs by the intravenous route.

INFECTION CONTROL

Patients receiving intravenous therapy seem particularly suscep-tible to nosocomial infection. Since this problem is great, the Center for Disease Control in Atlanta issued a list of recommendations for reduc-ing the incidence of infection in 1973.

It is most important that these recommendations be adhered to, since time-testing of the recommendations has resulted in a significant reduction of infection.

The agency's infections committee should approve all policies and procedures related to intravenous therapy. This serves to further con-trol infection.

WATCHDOGGING

The agency should have a "watchdog" attitude toward all personnel administering intravenous therapy. Watchdogging implies controlling who is allowed to be involved in the therapeutic plan. The agency should be so selective as to assign intravenous therapy duties only to those nurses who have demonstrated expertise.

Periodic on-site evaluations of the nurse's performance and evalua-tion of her or his knowledge base is recommended.

ADMINISTRATION OF DRUGS AS RECOMMENDED

Medications should be administered only after careful review of the literature and utilization of the recommended methods for reconstitu-tion and dilution.

Serious side effects occur when medications of too high or low con-centrations are administered. The drug may become ineffective, irri-tating, or lethal.

Should physicians insist on ordering medications to be given in con-centrations contrary to what is recommended, it is advisable to obtain a signed statement from that physician confirming the safety of the altered method. Final approval rests with the P and T committee.

Should the nurse's judgment contradict any altered method, she or he has the right to refuse to perform the function.

INTRAVENOUS (IV) TEAMS

Intravenous (IV) teams are composed of registered nurses who are trained to deliver all aspects of IV therapy. Nurses on IV teams perform the duties of starting infusions and transfusions, administering IV push and piggyback medications, administering IV site care, and assessing, planning, implementing, and evaluating conditions related to the ther-apy and its complications.

The Center for Disease Control recommends the use of IV teams when possible, since this specialization affords a closer and continuous watchdog where infection control is concerned.

The major advantage of the IV team is expertise. The same pair of eyes can best see changes in the patient's condition from day to day. It is by performing the same task repetitiously that one becomes expert in its performance.

Health care delivery is most effective when a multidisciplinary approach is used. In intravenous therapy the nurse may be advisor to the pharmacist regarding clinical practice and the pharmacist may be

INTRAVENOUS FLUID SCHEDULE Form 5232–Rev. 6-73

FLOOR DATE OCHSNER FOUNDATION HOSPITAL

ROOM	PATIENT NAME	✓ IF PRE-OP	FLUID ORDERED (KIND & AMT.) MEDICATION ADDED, START, RESTART, ADD TYPE OF NEEDLE IF ORDERED	RATE	TIME REQUEST PLACED	NURSE	VENIPUNCTURE SITE & TYPE NEEDLE USED	TIME STARTED	IV NURSE

TYPE & MATCH

ROOM	PATIENT NAME	T & M, T & H, COOMBS	TIME REQUEST PLACED	NURSE	IV NURSE

DRESSING CHANGES

ROOM	PATIENT NAME	TIME	SUBCLAVIAN	SORENSEN	JELCO	BUTTERFLY	OTHER	I. V. NURSE AND/OR COMMENTS

Fig. 1-1. IV fluid schedule sheet is posted in each nursing unit. Unit nurse posts therapy to be administered: infusions, transfusions, IV push and piggyback medications, site care, and blood specimens to be collected. IV nurse notes and signs care done when procedure(s) is completed.

advisor to the nurse on pharmacotherapeutics and pharmacodynamics. The nurse may have an equal exchange with blood bank personnel.

The unit nurse may have the responsibility of preparing all medications, fluids, and equipment prior to initiation of IV therapy by the IV nurse. In most agencies where IV teams are utilized, all preparation and administration is carried out by the IV nurse. The pharmacist is usually responsible for admixing all infusions and piggyback medications.

In order to function effectively, two to four IV nurses are required for each 50 infusions to be started. Since most infusions are initiated on the day tour of duty, the number of nurses required for the second half of the evening and the night tour of duty may be reduced. When IV push and piggyback therapy is a function of the unit nurse, the number of IV nurses may be further reduced.

IV nurses make rounds on each patient care unit at the beginning, middle, and end of each tour of duty. This is done to assess, plan, implement, and evaluate their charge. The team is notified by the unit nurse for unscheduled procedures.

An IV fluid schedule sheet (Fig. 1-1) may be used by the unit nurse to schedule routine and special procedures. The sheet may also serve as a source for documentation of care delivered by the IV nurse. In such cases the IV fluid schedule sheet is maintained as a legal document.

IV nurses are specialists in their field and as such play a vital role in the care of patients receiving intravenous therapy.

References

Alton Ochsner Medical Foundation, Hospital Division, Department of Nursing Service: Policy manual, New Orleans, 1977, The Foundation.

American Nurses' Association: Code for professional nurses, ANA publ. code no. G-56, Kansas City, Mo., 1976.

Center for Disease Control: Recommendations for the prevention of IV associated infections, Atlanta, 1973, Bacterial Diseases Branch, Bureau of Epidemiology.

Creighton, H.: Changing legal attitudes: the effect of the law on nursing, publ. no. 20-1212, New York, 1974, National League for Nursing.

Gentry, J.: Excerpts from a collection of papers on the legal responsibilities of the nurse, New Orleans, 1973, Alton Ochsner Medical Foundation, Hospital Division, Department of Nursing Service.

Lesnik, M., and Anderson, B.: Nursing practice and the law, ed. 2, Philadelphia, 1963, J. B. Lippincott Co.

Primm, M.: L.S.N.A. gives views on IV therapy to board of nursing, Pelican News **34:** 1, Spring 1978.

Chapter 2

Infection control

Infection is listed among the inherent dangers of intravenous therapy. Contaminated intravenous systems, sites, fluids, and medications may produce serious infections with resulting ill effects to the patient.

Particulate matter is described as a foreign substance present within the intravenous system. This material includes metal, rubber, plastic, glass, paper fibers, molds, cotton fibers, and drug particles. When particulate matter enters the patient, infection, granulomas, or other complications may ensue.

Airborne bacteria, bags, bottles, tubings, needles, cannulae, fluids, medications, outdated equipment, glass ampules, tourniquets, the patient's skin, tape, dressings, and the therapist are all sources of contamination. Virtually anything coming in contact with the patient that is unsterile or that may have been inadvertently contaminated is considered dangerous.

In addition, contamination may result from breaks in the closed system such as when intravenous push or piggyback medications are administered through punctures in reseal injection sites.

The causative organisms include gram-positive and gram-negative bacteria (predominant organisms are *Serratia*, *Klebsiella*, and *Pseudomonas*) and fungi (predominantly *Candida albicans*).

Specific infection control and prevention measures must be practiced in order that the complications of intravenous therapy can be prevented or minimized.

Concern over this nosocomial infection was so great during the 1970s that the Center for Disease Control (CDC) and physicians and agencies in authority issued specific recommendations for infection control.

Measures used to control infection are to be applied during initiation and maintenance of intravenous therapy.

17

Infection control techniques for total parenteral nutrition and blood therapy are included at the end of this chapter.

INFECTION CONTROL PRACTICES RELATED TO INITIATION OF THERAPY
Bags and bottles

In the selection and preparation of equipment, collapsible, unvented fluid bags that use the closed system principle are preferred to vented, open-system type bottles.

Fluid bottles with unfiltered vents allow air to enter the bottle as the fluid flows out, permitting airborne bacteria to enter. In addition, when the IV tubing is connected to the bottle, some fluid may leak out of the bottle and remain on the bottle lip. When the bottle is inverted and the drip chamber squeezed, this contaminated fluid backflows into the bottle. Minimize backflow by squeezing the drip chamber of the IV tubing before inserting it into the bottle.

Inspect fluid containers prior to use. Do not use faulty containers such as those with cracks, leaks, and cloudy or precipitated fluid. Return faulty containers to the manufacturer for investigation. Discard outdated fluids. Avoid using bottles that have lost their vacuum.

Medication preparation

Only experienced personnel should admix medications. Use the agency's admixture service whenever possible. Determine incompatibilities of drugs and diluents. If present, do not mix incompatible drugs and fluids.

Vein irritation of the chemical type can be prevented or minimized by compatibility determinations and utilization of fluids that are as near neutral in pH as possible. Cortisone preparations or sodium bicarbonate are sometimes added to fluids in minimal dosages to reduce vein irritation.

The possibility of cross contamination may be appreciably reduced when single-dose vials and ampules of diluents are drugs are used in preparing medications for admixture or direct administration.

Tubing preparation

Once an IV tubing is connected to the fluid container and primed or bled of air, an additional 30 to 50 ml of fluid should be allowed to flow through the tubing. This fluid removes most particulate matter from the tubing. This flushing fluid is discarded. Most commercial fluids have an extra 50 ml of fluid in each container for this purpose as well as to allow for waste. Therefore there is little danger of short-changing the patient of a prescribed amount of fluid.

Closed-system maintenance

A closed system in IV therapy indicates that there is a seal between the fluid container, the IV tubing, the needle or cannula, and the patient.

In most cases it is impossible to keep the system closed; however, certain measures can be used to minimize breaks in the system. These include avoidance of repeated needle punctures into reseal injection sites and flash chambers and avoidance of using three-way stopcocks.

When adding fluid containers to in-progress infusions, clamp the IV tubing as close to its end as possible.

Handwashing

Handwashing, when adhered to, can significantly reduce the incidence of nosocomial infections. This applies to all phases of patient care.

It is recommended that hands be washed before and after each procedure. A soap containing a suitable anti-infective agent should be used.

Gloving and draping

The CDC recommends that following handwashing, sterile gloves should be donned and the site draped prior to starting infusions and during IV site care. This is the ideal and in many instances is practiced. The practicality of such a measure of infection control is questioned by some.

Needles and cannulae

Selection of the needle or cannula is based on the length of therapy, condition of the veins, and the viscosity and irritating potential of the fluid and medication to be administered.

The incidence of mechanical and chemical vein irritation and inflammation can be reduced when the needle or cannula is of a size smaller than the vein.

Stainless steel needles should be utilized whenever possible, since the incidence of phlebitis and fungal overgrowth is less frequent than when plastic devices are used.

Site preparation

Site preparation begins with evaluation of the condition of the skin and veins. Areas of phlebitis, sclerosis, inflammation, and skin breaks from previous therapy or other conditions should be avoided.

Should the patient have a large quantity of body hair, it should be clipped, as opposed to shaved, since shaving creates microabrasions that predispose the area to infection (Maki et al., 1973). Depilatory

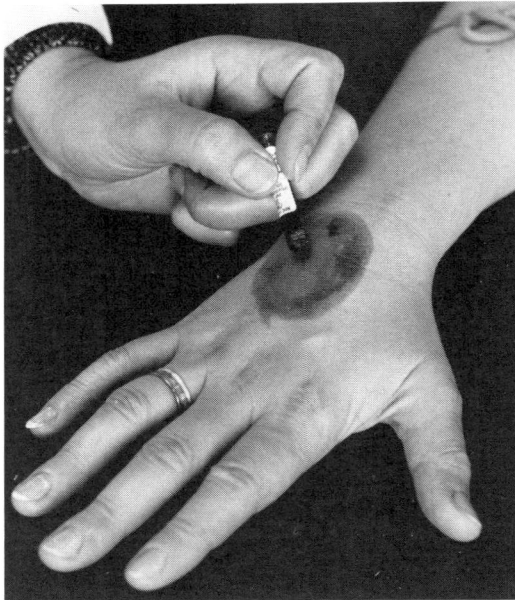

Fig. 2-1. Cleansing of IV site. IV site should be vigorously scrubbed using friction and circular motion. Scrub from center of site out to 5 cm (2 inch) periphery. (Courtesy Alton Ochsner Medical Foundation, New Orleans.)

agents are sometimes used, although the possibility of allergic reactions and skin irritation is present.

Following the removal of excessive hair the site is cleansed. The most effective anti-infective agents are tincture of iodine, 1% or 2% iodine in 70% alcohol, povidone iodine, or other iodophors (CDC 1973).

Should tincture of iodine be used, it should be removed with 70% isopropyl alcohol after the iodine dries on the skin.

If the patient is allergic to these anti-infectives, 70% isopropyl alcohol can be used.

The IV site should be vigorously scrubbed using friction and a circular motion (Fig. 2-1). The scrub should be done for 1 minute and allowed to dry for 30 to 60 seconds. Scrub from the center of the site out to a 5 cm (2 inch) periphery.

Taping

Excessive movement of the needle or cannula within the skin and vein can have a mechanically irritating and inflaming effect. Once venipuncture is performed, the needle or cannula should be taped in such a way as to minimize to-and-fro motion.

Water-repellant tape should be used to assure adhesiveness and dryness of the area involved.

Antimicrobial ointments

Antimicrobial ointments, when applied at the time of insert and every 24 hours for the duration of the therapy, will significantly reduce the incidence of bacterial and fungal overgrowth at the IV site.

Antibiotic ointments are not recommended, since the invading organisms usually resist their effects.

Dressings

Dry, sterile, occlusive dressings applied over the IV site will aid in preventing the entrance of contaminants.

A dressing is applied at the time the IV is inserted. It is changed every 24 hours thereafter for the duration of the therapy.

Dressings are labeled with the date and time of application. The date and time of insertion, the size and type of needle or cannula used, and the therapist's name should be included on the label.

Filters

The use of in-line and syringe type filters of the 0.45 μm and 0.22 μm size is recommended. Filters remove particulate matter, bacteria, fungi, and air from the IV system. Studies reveal that the 0.45 μm filter removes all bacteria, fungi, and particulate matter for up to 6 to 8 hours, after which fungi and some bacteria, particularly *Pseudomonas* escape. The 0.22 μm filter removes all of the aforementioned particles and contaminants for up to 72 hours. Total wetting of filters with the IV fluid removes air and promotes maximum filtration.

Laminar flow hoods

Virtually 100% of all airborne bacteria is removed from the air by the laminar flow system. Outside air is drawn into the system by vacuum and filtered. This filtered air is then jetted to a specified work area in uniform streams (Fig. 2-2).

All equipment used to prepare IV fluids and medications is placed in the work area in rows. This allows the uniform streams of air to continue their flow.

Once the IV fluid or medication is prepared, it is removed from the work area and taken to the patient care area.

Since the air within the work area is considered free of airborne bacteria, the possibility of introducing contaminants into the fluid or medication is greatly reduced (Abbott, 1970).

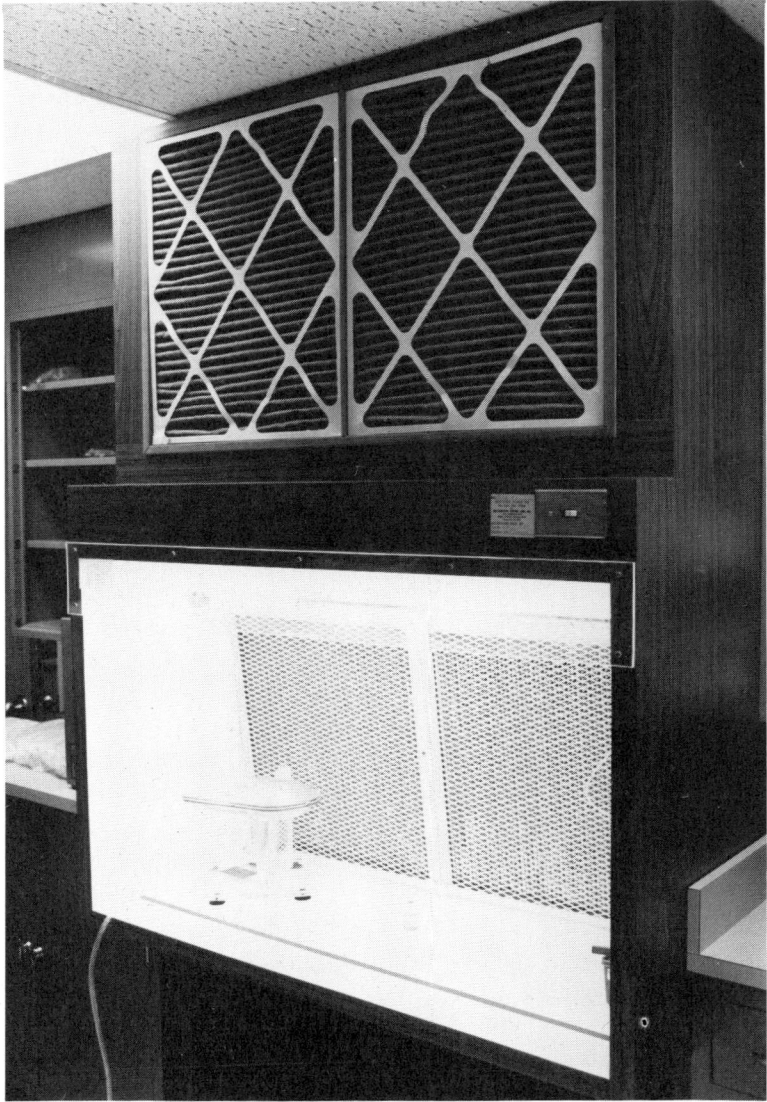

Fig. 2-2. Laminar flow hood. Outside air is drawn into system by vacuum and filtered. This filtered air is then jetted to work area in uniform streams. (Courtesy Alton Ochsner Medical Foundation, New Orleans.)

INFECTION CONTROL PRACTICES RELATED TO MAINTENANCE OF THERAPY

Inspection

Monitoring day-to-day changes in the condition of the patient and the IV site requires a skilled observer. The use of IV teams affords the opportunity for the same pair of eyes to observe for changes.

The very first sign of inflammation, phlebitis, pain, or pyogenesis warrants immediate discontinuation of the infusion.

Signs of systemic infection or pyrogenic reactions, septicemia, bacteremia, and fungemia such as fever, chills, diaphoresis, hypotension, and gastrointestinal or neurologic symptoms warrant discontinuation of the infusion and culture of the fluid, tubing, needle, or cannula and the patient's blood.

Site care

Daily site care is essential (Fig. 2-3). This can be accomplished by removing the previous dressing, defatting and cleansing the skin with acetone and povidone iodine or 70% isopropyl alcohol, application of a suitable antimicrobial ointment, and a dry, sterile, occlusive dressing. The dressing should be labeled as previously recommended.

Maintenance of equipment

IV bags or bottles and tubings, including extension tubings, should be changed every 24 hours. Studies reveal that contamination of this equipment and fluid by an overgrowth of pathogenic and nonpathogenic organisms after this time period increases.

Use of 250 ml containers of fluid for keep-open infusions provides incentive for changing these containers every 24 hours.

Site rotation

Ideally, IV sites should be rotated every 48 to 72 hours. The condition of the patient and availability of veins may prevent this. Site rotation aids in minimizing the incidence of phlebitis and related complications.

Studies indicate that some form of infection occurs when IVs are allowed to continue beyond the 72-hour period even with scrupulous adherence to infection control practices.

Treatment and prevention of complications

Dependent and independent nursing actions are employed in treating complications related to intravenous infections.

Discontinue infusions and restart at other sites. Antibiotics and antifungal agents may be administered. Treat areas of phlebitis by apply-

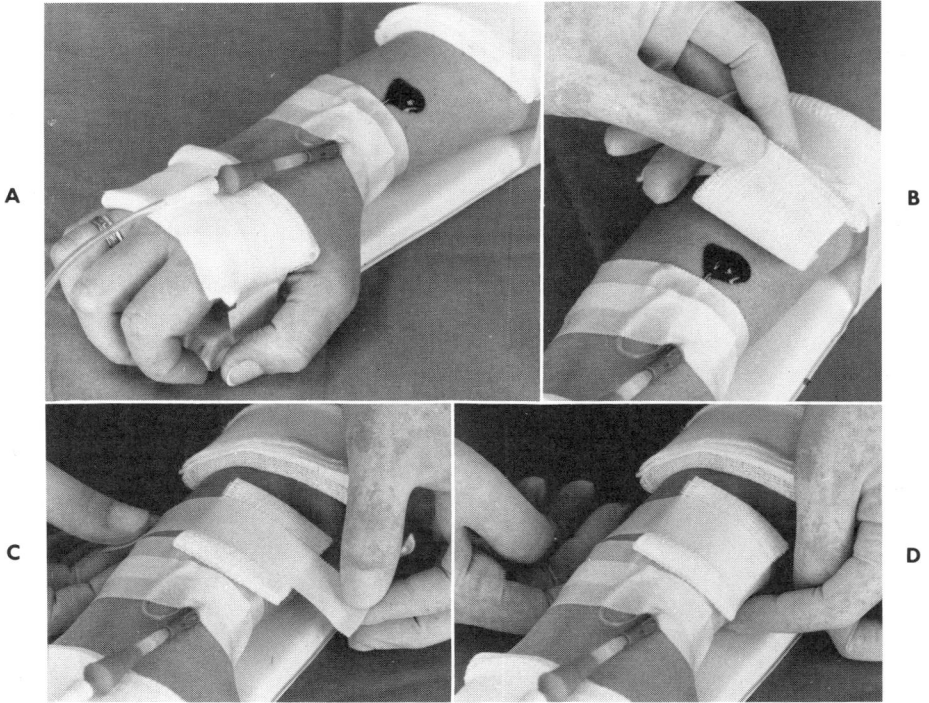

Fig. 2-3. IV site care. **A,** Following removal of previous dressing, defatting and cleansing skin with acetone and povidone iodine or 70% isopropyl alcohol, a suitable antimicrobial ointment is applied to IV site. **B,** A dry, sterile dressing is applied to IV site. **C** and **D,** Taping of dry, sterile dressing at IV site. (Courtesy Alton Ochsner Medical Foundation, New Orleans.)

ing warm, moist compresses to the site for 20 to 30 minutes, four times a day.

As a rule, IV therapy should be initiated and continued for only as long as absolutely necessary.

SPECIFIC INFECTION CONTROL TECHNIQUES RELATED TO TOTAL PARENTERAL NUTRITION (TPN)

Experienced personnel who utilize a laminar flow hood are to prepare all TPN solutions.

Refrigerate solutions prepared in advance at 4 C (39.2 F).

TPN solutions are highly concentrated dextrose solutions and contain protein that is known to be incompatible with many substances. As such it is important to avoid IV push and piggyback administration of other substances by way of this solution.

Cannula insertion is considered a surgical procedure because of the location of the subclavian vein. Strict asepsis is vital, since the cannula is most often kept in place for several weeks. The hair around the site is shaved and the skin prepared utilizing principles of surgical asepsis.

The physician inserting the cannula and the physician's assistant should wear surgical caps, masks, gowns, and gloves during the procedure. Sterile draping of the area is required.

Dressings at subclavian sites are occlusive in nature and are changed every 24 to 48 hours. Should a dressing become moist or contaminated, more frequent changes are indicated.

Should complications such as fever or glucose intolerance develop, the entire system should become suspect. Removal and culturing of the suspect system may be indicated. The infusion site may be altered at this time using an entirely new system.

Tubing and bags should be changed every 8 to 12 hours (usual time for infusing one unit).

Use of intralipids in TPN is advantageous, since replacement of some glucose with fat reduces the tonicity of the TPN solution. Another advantage of intralipid therapy is that this solution can be administered peripherally with a stainless steel needle.

SPECIFIC INFECTION CONTROL TECHNIQUES
RELATED TO BLOOD THERAPY

Because of rigid rules and regulations related to blood therapy, the incidence of infection is much less frequent than with other forms of IV therapy. Nevertheless, there are certain key points to be considered.

Blood should be administered within 30 minutes from the time it arrives from the blood bank. If administration is delayed, the blood should be returned to the bank for refrigeration.

Contamination of blood by overgrowth of organisms can begin anytime following the 30-minute time period.

There is a great chance of infection during the following platelet administration because platelets are pooled.

Malaria and hepatitis may occur but can be controlled by the changing of all tubings following blood administration.

References

Abbott Laboratories: IV additives: steps to safety, (Robert L. Ravin, collaborator), Chicago, 1970, Abbott Laboratories.

Center for Disease Control: Recommendations for the prevention of IV-associated infections, Atlanta, 1973, Bacterial Diseases Branch, Bureau of Epidemiology.

Francke, D.: Handbook of IV additive review, Drug intelligence publication, Hamilton, Ill., 1973, The Hamilton Press.

Maki, D. G., Goldman, D. A., and Rhame, F. S.: Infection control in intravenous therapy, Ann. Intern. Med. **79**:867, 1973.

Chapter 3

Techniques of intravenous therapy

Success rates with the minimization of complications in intravenous therapy are attributed to the use of techniques that carry with them scientific principles.

The actual performance of most aspects of intravenous therapy is simple. It is easy to train one to start, regulate, and discontinue infusions, and to reconstitute, dilute, and administer medications. However, the art of placing intravenous therapy in the perspectus of a science is complex.

Intravenous therapy is a frequently administered treatment. Approximately 25% of all patients admitted to today's acute care setting receive some form of intravenous therapy during their stay in the institution.

Complications, although not always life-threatening, pose a threat to the patient, and apprehension on the part of the patient may interfere with his or her acceptance and resultant success of the therapy.

Certain key factors related to the techniques of intravenous therapy are considered in this chapter. Consideration is given to the anatomy and physiology of the integumentary, circulatory, and nervous systems; the psychological and physical preparation of the patient; the procedures involved in initiating the therapy; the equipment used; and general information concerning maintenance of therapy. Hypodermoclysis is also included.

ANATOMY AND PHYSIOLOGY

A review of the structure and function of the integumentary and circulatory systems can be of value to the nurse performing intravenous therapy.

The skin, composed of two layers called epidermis and dermis, serves as a barrier or the body's first line of defense from the outside world.

Breaks in the skin by irritating forces or invaders such as needles and cannulae can produce harmful effects on the body as a whole.

A unique structural feature of the dermis is the arrangement of the cells of its first layer. The arrangement is in parallel rows of small papillae that attach the epidermis to the dermis. In addition, the dermis contains many elastic fibers that account for the extensibility and elasticity of the skin. During the aging process the numbers of elastic fibers decrease as does the amount of subcutaneous fat (Anthony, 1979).

Skin texture is determined by such factors as age, color, and states of hydration. Skin elasticity lessens through the aging process and in the presence of certain disease processes.

Skin color is determined by deposits of a pigment called melanin. The larger the deposit of melanin, the darker and, in some cases, the tougher the skin will be.

When appropriately stimulated, the skin's heat and cold receptors produce either vasodilation or vasoconstriction.

A sheath of areolar connective tissue called the subcutaneous or superficial fascia attaches the dermis to the underlying structures. Beneath this lies a layer of fibrous tissue called the deep fascia, which covers the muscles, forms partitions between the muscles, attaches some muscle to bone, and encloses viscera, glands, veins, arteries, and nerves. Although varying amounts of fat are deposited in the superficial fascia, the deep fascia contains no fat. It is in the superficial fascia that the superficial veins are located. The amount of underlying tissue present does have bearing on successful needle or cannula placement and maintence, since the amount and condition of the underlying tissue has a direct effect on the condition of the vein.

Nerves and nerve fibers vary in their distribution and, as such, certain portions of the skin are more sensitive than others. As an example, the anterior forearm is more sensitive than is the posterior forearm.

The circulatory system, first described by William Harvey, is composed of the lung, heart, veins, arteries, capillaries, blood, bone marrow, and venous sinuses. This system is also divided into the pulmonary and systemic portions.

The pulmonary portion is composed of the right ventricle of the heart, pulmonary artery, lungs, pulmonary veins, and left atrium and left ventricle of the heart.

The systemic portion is composed of the aorta, arteries, arterioles, capillaries, venules, and veins (Plumer, 1975). It is the systemic portion that is of greater concern to the nurse performing intravenous therapy.

Blood flow within the circulatory system takes the following course: aorta to arteries to arterioles to venules (capillaries) to veins to vena cavae to right atrium through the tricuspid valve to right ventricle to pulmonary artery and its semilunar valve to the lungs to pulmonary veins to left atrium through the bicuspid valve (mitral) to left ventricle to aorta.

Normal circulation time is approximately 18 to 24 seconds. Circulation time may decrease in anemia and hyperthyroidism and increase in hypertension, myxedema, and cardiac failure (Thomas, 1977).

Alterations in circulation time are to be considered, since the onset of action of medications and effectiveness of certain other phases of intravenous therapy may vary accordingly.

Arteries and veins are composed of three layers of tissue. These layers are called tunica intima (inner layer), tunica media (middle layer), and tunica adventitia (outer layer).

The tunica intima of both arteries and veins is composed of an elastic and smooth endothelial lining. Within large veins this endothelial tissue forms semilunar folds or valves that assist blood as it circulates back to the heart. A noticeable bulge, usually at bifurcations of superficial veins, many times indicates the presence of a valve.

Valves within veins may interfere with withdrawal of blood. When suction is applied the valves compress and tend to collapse the vein. Needle or cannula adjustment usually remedies this problem.

In cases of phlebitis or thrombosis, smaller veins can be used, since they contain no valves. The needle or cannula can be inserted in a distal direction, allowing for flow of an intravenous fluid or medication in an opposite direction. Eventually the infused substance will reach an unaffected vein and flow in a proximal direction (Plumer, 1975).

The tunica media of arteries and veins is composed of muscular and elastic tissue and vasoconstrictive and vasodilative nerve fibers. Impulses to constrict or dilate come from the medulla oblongata. The arterial tunica media generally remains in a tonus state, while the tunica media of veins tends to collapse as pressure within the vessel rises or falls. The musculature within the tunica media of veins is weaker than in arteries.

Temperature changes and irritation produce spasms in both arteries and veins. The application of heat may relieve spasms and its associated pain and promote circulation.

The tunica adventitia of arteries and veins is composed of areolar connective tissue. This tissue surrounds and supports the vessels. The tunica adventitia of arteries is thicker than that of veins. Greater strength of arteries is required because of greater pressure within these vessels (Plumer, 1975).

Arteries are generally deep and protected by muscle. Occasionally an artery is superficially located and as such is called aberrant (Adriani, 1962).

Arterial puncture should be restricted to the injection of radiopaque dyes for x-ray and other related diagnostic procedures, collection of arterial blood for blood gas determination, and in some instances administration of certain medications.

Deep arteries and veins are generally enclosed in the same sheath of fascia. An abnormal opening between an artery and vein can develop through a congenital abnormality or through trauma. This abnormal opening is called an arteriovenous fistula or anastomosis (Guyton, 1976; Plumer, 1975).

Within the anastomosis blood flows directly into the vein, decreasing peripheral resistance. The vein becomes overburdened by this extra and high-pressured flow of blood. The involved vein is usually large and tortuous, making venipuncture difficult.

An arteriovenous fistula or anastomosis is many times surgically created for the purpose of hemodialysis.

The distinct difference in veins and arteries lies in the composition, capacity, numbers, and presence of valves.

The ability to distinguish veins from arteries is far more important than is knowledge of names of veins and arteries. Puncture and the inadvertent injection of certain medications into arteries can lead to complications such as irritation, necrosis, sloughing, and in some instances gangrene and loss of function of the affected part (Adriani, 1962). One method for distinguishing veins from arteries is by checking for pulsation. If it pulsates, it is an artery.

There are three sets of veins: the superficial or subcutaneous found between layers of superficial fascia and immediately between skin layers; the deep veins that lie side by side with arteries and that are usually enclosed in the same sheath; and the venous sinuses found only in the anterior skull.

The superficial veins are those of greatest concern to the nurse performing venipuncture. Venous sinuses are rarely used in intravenous therapy because of the dangers of infection and osteomyelitis and therefore will not be discussed in this text.

Deep veins usually accompany an artery and nerve. These may lie side by side or in close proximity. This is not always true with superficial veins.

Deep veins sometimes unite with superficial veins. This union is most commonly found in the veins of the lower extremities. Because of this, a thrombus occurring within a superficial vein of the lower extremity may extend to one of the deep veins of that extremity, causing

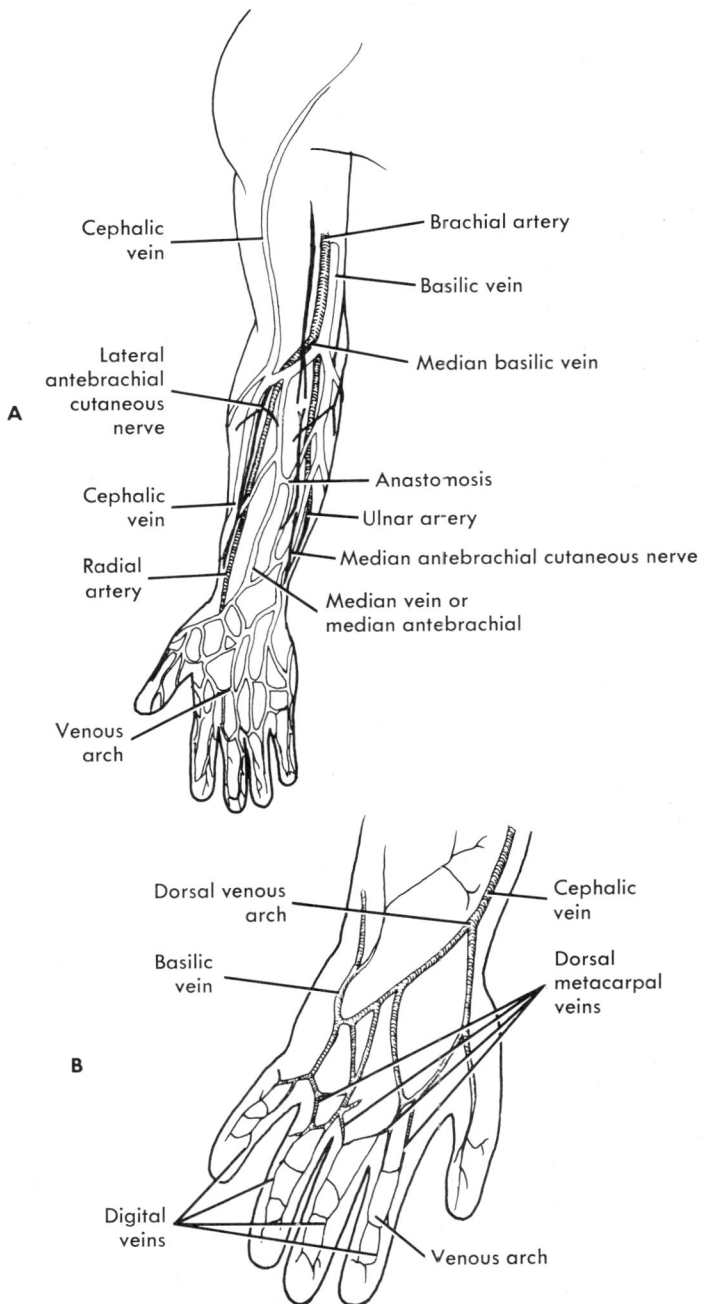

Fig. 3-1. A to **C,** Significant superficial veins of upper extremities, neck, and trunk. (**C** from Anthony, C. P., and Thibodeau, G. A.: Textbook of anatomy and physiology, ed. 10, St. Louis, 1979, The C. V. Mosby Co.)

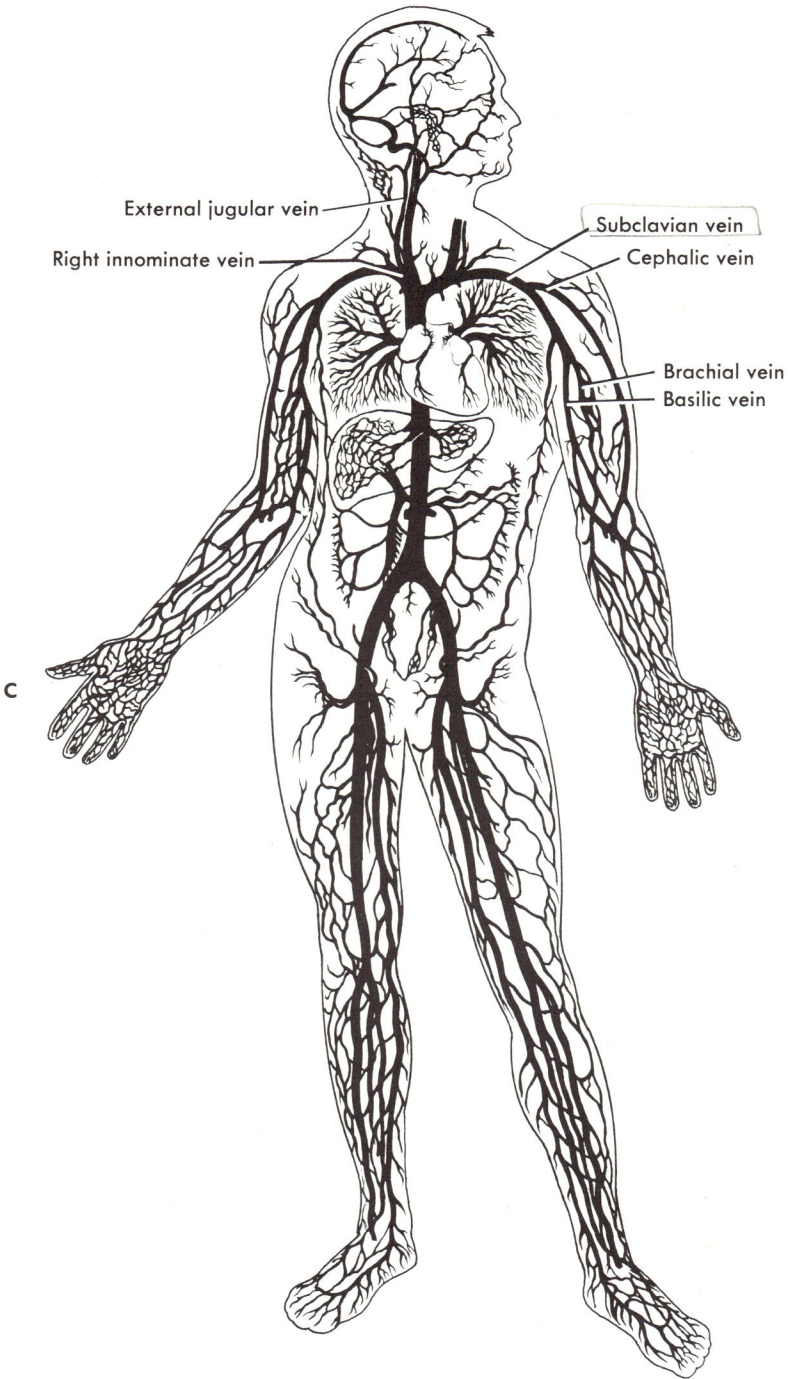

External jugular vein

Right innominate vein

Subclavian vein

Cephalic vein

Brachial vein

Basilic vein

C

Fig. 3-1, cont'd. For legend see opposite page.

a pulmonary embolism. It is recommended that veins of the lower extremities be avoided (Plumer, 1975).

Varicosed veins should be avoided, since stasis and stagnation of blood in these veins is common due to loss of muscle tone and inadequate circulation of blood. Medications administered in these veins can pool, thereby weakening the effect of the medication. Later, this same medication may begin to circulate and could lead to a drug overdosage.

Irritating chemicals administered can injure all layers of a vein, causing a sterile inflammation. This condition is called phlebothrombosis or phlebitis with secondary thrombosis. Prolonged irritation from any cause can render the vessel useless for therapy.

Thrombophlebitis is inflammation of a vein developing before the formation of an obvious thrombosis (Thomas, 1977).

Thrombophlebitis indicates vein inflammation and clot formation, while phlebothrombosis indicates clot formation and nonobvious phlebitis (Plumer, 1975).

Neck veins form dorsal and venous arches and, along with a network of superficial veins of the lower arm, drain into two larger veins—the cephalic and basilic veins.

Fig. 3-1 shows the significant superficial veins of the upper extremities, neck, and trunk. These veins include the digital, metacarpal, cephalic, basilic, and medial veins.

PATIENT PREPARATION
Psychologic preparation

Patients' immediate response to intravenous therapy varies according to the type of treatment they are to receive.

With infusions they may feel that their condition is critical. These feelings usually stem from previous experiences and tales of woe they may have heard from significant others. Those who have experienced multiple punctures may be "needle shy."

With transfusion, patients may experience feelings of despair. They may feel that their condition is grave. Since hemorrhage and shock may be present at this time, feelings of anxiety may well be warranted because the condition of the patient may indeed be critical.

With intravenous push medications by way of intermittent devices a patient's fear may be less pronounced although certain fears may still prevail.

A therapeutic nurse-patient relationship should be initiated prior to beginning intravenous therapy. The establishment of rapport and an effective system of communication should be of utmost concern to the nurse. It is appropriate to utilize the nursing process in performing any phase of intravenous therapy.

Assessment of probable and possible response is based on a patient's knowledge, prior responses to therapy, and mental and physical state.

Planning the care should include the nurses' preparation for the administration of the procedure as well as instructing the patient with appropriate follow-up regarding the patient's interpretation of the instructions.

Implementation of the therapy should begin only after the patient has exhibited signs of understanding and acceptance.

Patient response should be evaluated following the initiation of therapy and each day thereafter unless conditions indicate more frequent evaluations.

Physical preparation

Prior to starting a continuous infusion, procedures such as hygiene, ambulation, enemas, and x-rays should be completed unless the therapy is classified as first priority.

All personal articles and the call bell should be within the patient's reach.

Instructions as to restrictions and limitations should be given. Included here are methods of ambulating with a portable IV standard, the importance of not applying pressure to the IV site, of keeping the site dry during bathing, and of keeping the fluid container at an appropriate height.

Patients should be given an estimate regarding the duration of therapy.

An understanding of the need for specified flow rates may prevent adjustments of flow rates by the patient.

The patient should be advised to notify the nurse should he or she experience pain or other complications. This does not discount the nurse's utilization of observations for signs and symptoms of complications.

The patient and significant others should be allowed to participate in the care he is receiving. Informing the patient cannot be overemphasized. Taking a few extra minutes to inform the patient helps the patient to understand what is happening. Countless minutes are saved in the long run.

CRITERIA FOR SITE SELECTION

Success or failure in intravenous therapy depends in part on the assessment and analysis of all factors that increase or decrease the possibility of success (Newman, 1952).

The first step in selecting a vein for continuous or intermittent infusions is to assess both hands and arms. A vein over a naturally splinted area should be the first choice, since this facilitates mobility. Such veins are located in the anterior and posterior forearm, the posterior hand, and the lateral upper arm. When possible the nondominant upper extremity should be used.

Jointed areas are avoided, since the infusion would render the part immobile and joint stiffness and pain would soon develop. Should a patient inadvertently exercise the joint, the needle or cannula may dislodge, puncture the vein, cause infiltration of the infusing substance, and perhaps damage the underlying tissue and nerves.

Choose a vein that will accommodate the needle or cannula to be used and one that will allow for free flow of the substance to be administered.

Superficial veins are preferred, since they are usually visible and palpable. It should be noted that the most visible and most palpable vein may not always be the best, since some may be occluded by sclerosis, giving them a ropelike texture. These veins may also be loosely connected, causing them to roll.

Rolling veins should not, however, present any great problem during venipuncture, providing that traction is applied distal to the puncture site. Traction temporarily anchors the vein so that the vein is immobile during puncture. Once entered, special taping may be required in order to prevent further rolling.

Thrombosed veins, varicosed veins, shunted areas, veins over joints and affected sides of radical mastectomy patient, and currently and previously traumatized and heavily scarred areas should be avoided unless otherwise indicated.

It is best to begin with distal veins and then work up, since previously damaged or injured proximal sites may present problems related to occlusion or extravasation. Extravasation of irritating substances at a previous punctured site proximal to the current site of puncture may cause necrosis and sloughing.

When irritating substances are administered, utilization of large veins is preferable, since greater dilution of the substance can be provided by the blood as it flows through these veins.

Should heat application be used to distend a vein, warm, moist heat applied to an entire part will promote greater circulation through vasodilation of the vessels.

When venipuncture is to be performed for the purpose of withdrawing blood or direct injection of a medication, the most suitable veins are those that lie within the antecubital fossa. The large diameter of these veins facilitates ease of insertion of relatively large needles or cannulae. There is also good support from underlying muscle and connective tissue. This serves to prevent rolling of these veins. Failure is kept at a minimum, since the possibility of vein collapse is miniscule. Smaller veins such as those located on the posterior hand present a different situation during withdrawal of blood. The size of these veins is smaller and there is less support from underlying muscle and connective tissue.

Veins within the antecubital fossa may be considered for infusions when no other vein is available, when situations are life-threatening, and when infusor-type flexible catheters are inserted.

When there is no arm vein available, the initiation of intravenous therapy becomes the responsibility of the physician, since nurses do not usually use other sites. Venous cutdowns (venisections) and puncturing of central veins are not considered to be within the scope of nursing practice.

The physician may choose to start the infusion in one of the superficial veins of the lower extremities, external jugular vein, subclavian vein, innominate vein, or to perform a venous cutdown (venisection).

It is recommended that veins of the lower extremities be avoided, since the possibility of complications such as thrombus formation outweigh the benefits.

Should the lower extremities be used, the following veins may be considered: veins at the ankle or dorsum of the foot, and those veins that course over the anterior and posterior medial and lateral malleolus.

In some agencies nurses are permitted to start infusions in sites other than the hands and arms. If so, the nurse should ascertain that this is included in the agency's policy and procedure on venipuncture and that training in this area is provided.

Two other important criteria for site selection is the patient's condition and the expected duration of therapy.

VENIPUNCTURE AND INTRAVENOUS INFUSION

Venipuncture may be performed for a variety of reasons. Patients are phlebotomized for the purpose of collecting blood samples for diagnostic study, collection of blood for autologous and recipient replacement, and removal of measured amounts of blood for the purpose of treating certain diseases such as idiopathic thrombocytopenia. Injections are performed for the purpose of administering one-time doses of medications; insertion of intermittent heparinized devices for administration of medications, infusions of water, nutrients, electrolytes, and medications over a prolonged period of time; infusion of fluid in minimal amounts for the purpose of keeping veins open in the event that they are needed for medication administration; blood transfusions; and crisis situations.

Equipment

The equipment needed for venipuncture varies according to the procedure to be performed. It is important to know what equipment will be needed and how the equipment functions in order that maximum effectiveness is obtained and that unnecessary complications are prevented.

The usual equipment needed includes needles and cannulae, intravenous fluid, medications, tubing, filters, tourniquets, tape, anti-infective agents, intravenous standards, and intravenous pumps and controllers.

The following discussion serves to provide information concerning the equipment used in intravenous therapy.

NEEDLES AND CANNULAE

Selection of the appropriate needle or cannula depends on the type and duration of therapy and the vein to be used.

Most needles are made of stainless steel while cannulae are made of plastic.

Since both carry with them certain advantages and disadvantages, it is appropriate to compare the two and examine each separately.

Cannulae

Plastics. Plastic cannulae are manufactured with polyvinyl chloride, Teflon, or silastic. They are coated with hemo-repellant material that assists in reducing thrombi formation on the catheter (Plumer, 1975).

Some studies reveal that vein irritation can be reduced by substituting the polyvinyl chloride type catheters with fluorethylene-propylene (Teflon). The fluorethylene-propylene substance is smooth textured with no graininess or roughness to add to catheter drag during insertion.

Most plastic cannulae are radiopaque. This is essential for verification of placement and location in case the catheter is lost in the patient.

Plastics are best for long-term therapy, when veins are few in number, and to assure that a vein will remain open.

There are two types of cannulae available: in-the-needle cannulae and over-the-needle cannulae (Nursing, 1972 survey).

In-the-needle cannulae. As the name suggests, the cannula rests inside the needle. The usual length of this type cannula is 4.5, 8, 9, 11.5, 21, 30, and 36 inches. The cannulae gauges are 14, 16, 17, 18, and 19.

The parts of the in-the-needle cannula include a trochar or stylet,

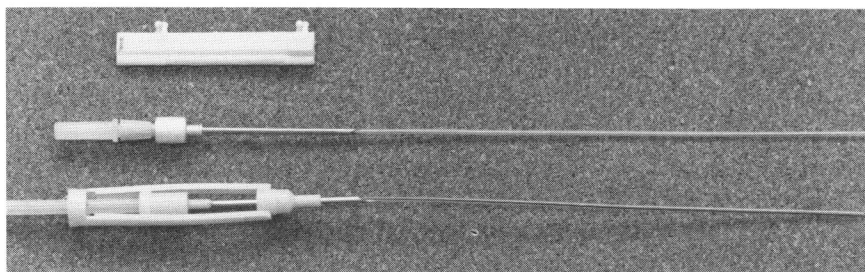

Fig. 3-2. In-the-needle type cannulae. Needle guard or protector is attached at junction of needle and cannula after insertion of cannula to prevent needle from severing plastic cannula. (Courtesy Alton Ochsner Medical Foundation, New Orleans.)

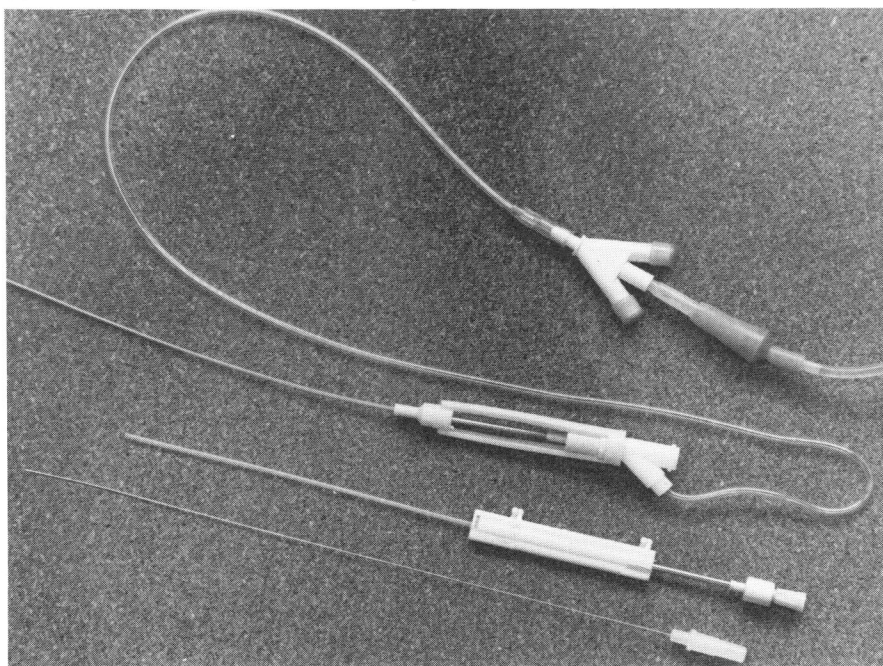

Fig. 3-3. In-the-needle type cannulae. Parts of in-the-needle cannula include trochar or stylet, cannula, needle protector, tubing, and, with some, a flash chamber. (Courtesy Alton Ochsner Medical Foundation, New Orleans.)

a cannula, needle protector, tubing, and sometimes a flash chamber (Figs. 3-2 and 3-3).

The in-the-needle cannula is used for central venous pressure monitoring, administration of total parenteral nutrition, and administration of other highly concentrated dextrose solutions. It is inserted into

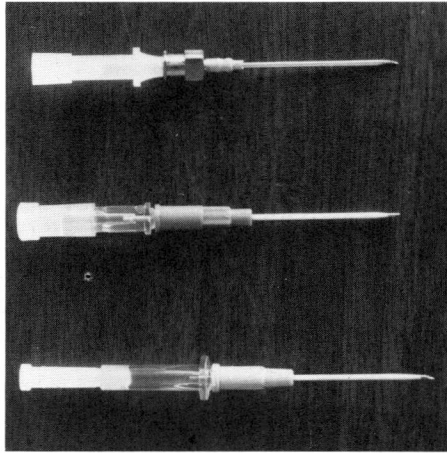

Fig. 3-4. Over-the-needle type cannulae. (Courtesy Alton Ochsner Medical Foundation, New Orleans.)

a large vein such as those in the antecubital fossa, the subclavian vein, or the jugular vein. Depending on the length of the cannula, it may be threaded from the entrance site into the right atrium of the heart.

Once inserted, cannulae of this type are secured in place with skin sutures.

Over-the-needle cannulae. As the name suggests, the cannula rests outside the needle (Fig. 3-4). Over-the-needle cannulae are 0.5, 2.25, 2.5, 5.5, 8, and 36 inches in length. The needle gauges are 14, 16, 18, 18.5, 20, and 22.

Over-the-needle cannulae of 0.5, 2.25, 2.5, 5, and 5.5 inches are commonly used for peripheral venipuncture. Insertion requires venipuncture and threading of the cannula over the needle and into the vein.

Threading requires pushing the catheter into the vein and pulling the needle outward simultaneously. It is important not to push the needle forward once the threading process begins, since there is a possibility that the catheter could be punctured or severed by the needle tip, creating a leak or causing a part of the catheter to break off and infuse into the patient.

Stainless steel needles

Needles utilized in intravenous therapy are made of stainless steel and are coated with silicone. This prevents corrosion, facilitates ease of insertion, and retards thrombi formation.

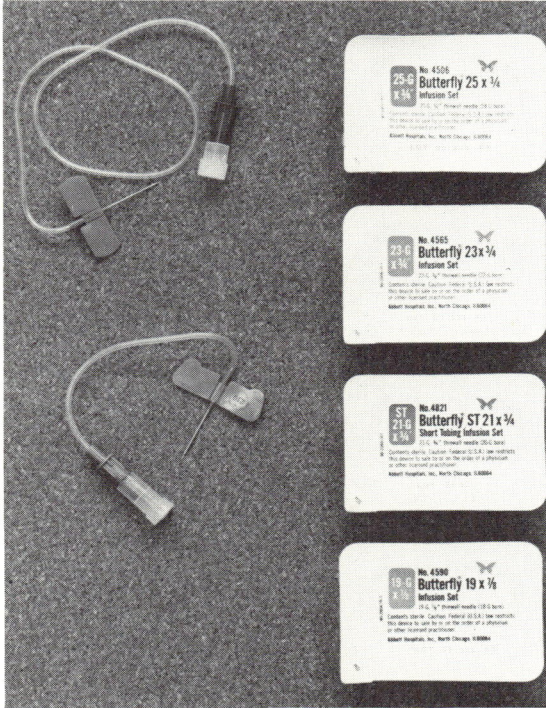

Fig. 3-5. Scalp vein or butterfly type needles with long and short tubings. (Courtesy Alton Ochsner Medical Foundation, New Orleans.)

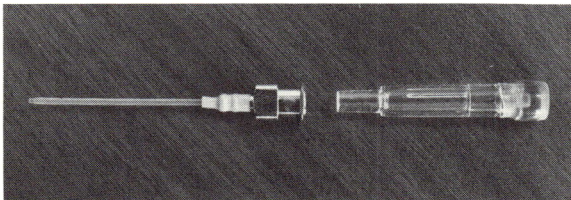

Fig. 3-6. Creation of heparin lock utilizing male adaptor plug and plastic over-the-needle cannula. (Courtesy Alton Ochsner Medical Foundation, New Orleans.)

Stainless steel needles are used for short-term and intermittent therapy.

According to the Center for Disease Control, stainless steel needles are preferred to plastic cannulae. Studies show a greater incidence of site infection with plastics, since there is a greater incidence of fungal overgrowth. Trauma to the vein is less severe with stainless steel than with plastic, since the needle gauge is smaller and the material is smoother.

The scalp vein or butterfly needle is more often preferred to a straight needle because it is easier to insert and because the scalp vein type needle has no hub, which could lead to further traumatization (Fig. 3-5).

The usual needle sizes are 12, 20, 21, 22, and 23 gauge.

Heparin locks or intermittent intravenous devices are scalp vein needles with a reseal injection site attached to the hard plastic tubing tip. Heparin locks can be created by attaching a male adaptor plug to the hub of most needles or cannulae (Fig. 3-6).

Needle gauge

Needle gauge refers to the inside and outside diameter of the lumen. Thin-walled needles indicate that the inside diameter of the lumen is thinner than usual. The advantage of using this type of needle is that the flow rate of fluid will be higher (Plumer, 1975).

Use of a short-beveled needle has certain advantages. The inferior vein wall is less likely to be punctured, the endothelial lining of the vein is less likely to be injured, the needle can most often be taped flat to the skin, there is lessened risk of hematoma when the needle enters the vein, and this type of needle is usually easier to insert.

Pain on insertion

It is not uncommon for the patient to experience slight to moderate pain on insertion of a needle or cannula. The larger the device the greater the pain. A local anesthetic such as plain lidocaine, 1% or 2%, may be used to infiltrate the IV site prior to venipuncture.

INTRAVENOUS FLUID

Once the prescribed intravenous fluid is selected, its container should be inspected for cracks or tears, foreign matter, cloudiness, precipitation, and any other sign of contamination. Should any of this be apparent, the fluid must not be used.

The fluid should be in date, and all medications added should be compatible.

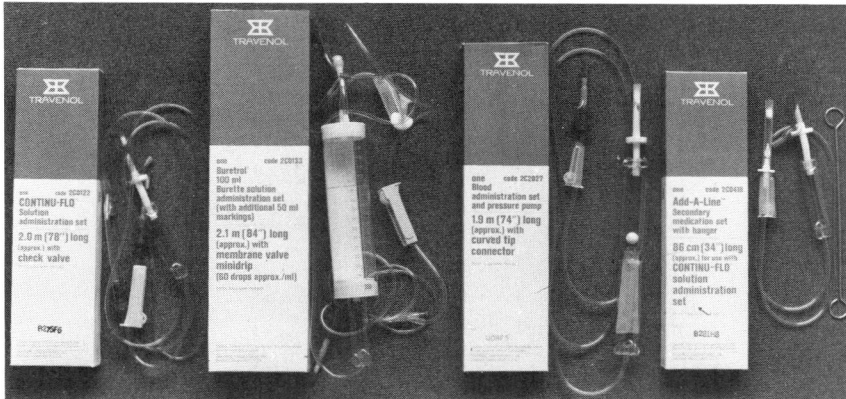

Fig. 3-7. Infusion tubing. (Courtesy Alton Ochsner Medical Foundation, New Orleans.)

All refrigerated fluid should be placed at room temperature for 30 to 60 minutes prior to being used.

The fluid container should be labeled with the patient's name and room number, drugs added and dosage, expiration date, name of admixer, and rate at which it is to be administered. The container should be waterclocked or time taped (Fig. 3-7).

MEDICATIONS

When medications are ordered to be added to infusions and when there is no admixture service provided by the pharmacy department, the nurse may have to add medications to infusion fluids. If so, the medications ordered should be reconstituted with the appropriate diluent and added to the infusion fluid. Strict aseptic technique must be practiced.

Verification of compatibility between medications and fluids is vital. Under no circumstances should incompatible substances be mixed together. Consultation with a pharmacist or the physician ordering the therapy may be necessary.

INTRAVENOUS TUBING

The appropriate intravenous tubing may be a regular solution administration set that delivers 10 to 15 drops/ml, a microdrop set of the burette type that delivers 60 drops/ml, or a straight or "Y" type blood administration set containing a regular or microaggregate filter (Fig. 3-8).

The choice of tubing and filter varies according to the therapy to

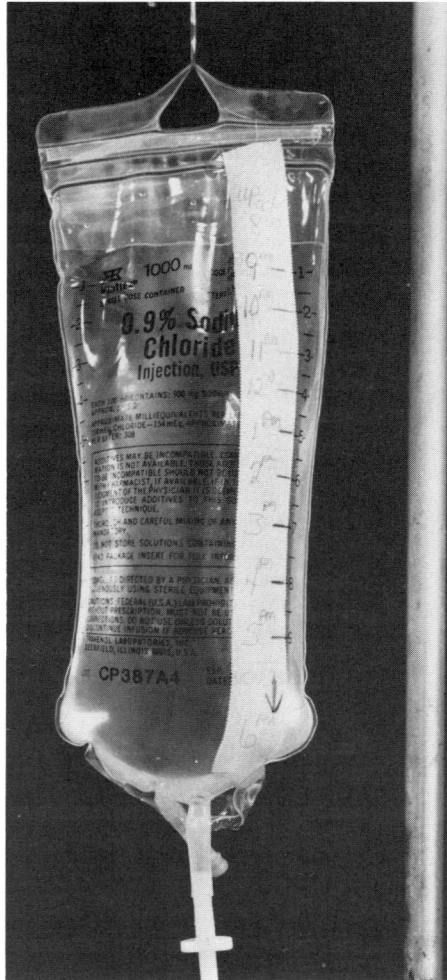

Fig. 3-8. Waterclocked fluid container. Medications-added label temporarily removed. (Courtesy Alton Ochsner Medical Foundation, New Orleans.)

be administered. Regular tubings are used for routine infusions and administration of intravenous piggyback medications; microdrop sets are used in pediatric and neonatal care and when relatively small amounts of fluid are to be administered over a relatively long period of time and when the infusion is to run at a keep-open rate; straight and "Y" type blood administration sets are used for blood administration and when blood administration is anticipated.

The microaggregate blood filter tubing is selected when it is anticipated that the patient will receive several units of blood. It is note-

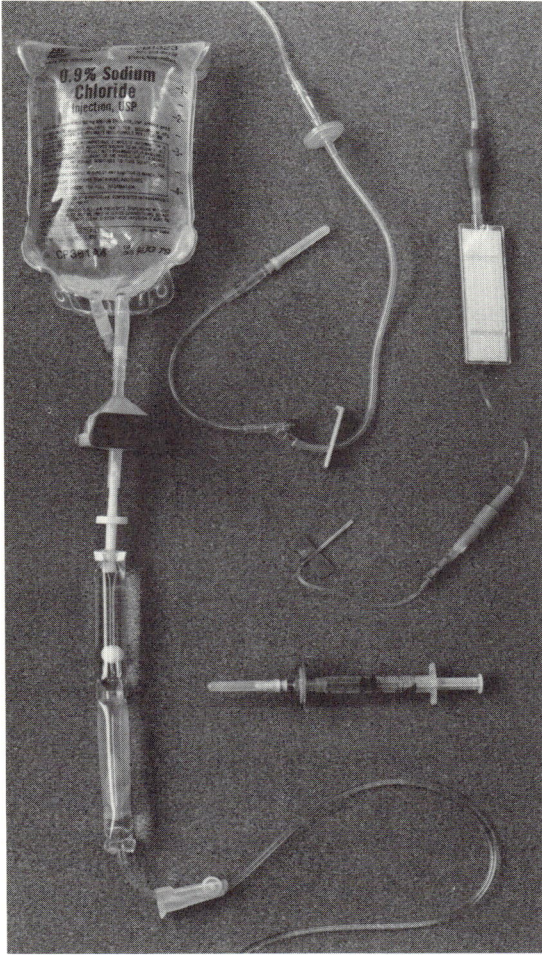

Fig. 3-9. Microaggregate, in-line, and syringe filters. (Courtesy Alton Ochsner Medical Foundation, New Orleans.)

worthy that current data advocates the use of microaggregate filters for all blood administration, since the filtration process is far superior to that obtained with regular blood administration sets. Time, cost, and patient benefits should be a consideration.

FILTERS

In-line filters of the 0.45 μm size will filter all bacteria, particulate matter, and air for 6 to 8 hours. Should the therapy extend beyond this time frame, a 0.22 μm filter should be used, since this size filter removes all bacteria, particulate matter, and air from the line for up to 72 hours (Fig. 3-9).

Extension tubes are attached to any of the aforementioned filters when the regular tubing length is inadequate, during surgical procedures when without an extension it would be difficult to administer substances without disturbing the sterile drape, and during total parenteral nutrition where the extension tube may serve as a safety mechanism against air embolism when the regular tubing is changed.

TOURNIQUETS

In order that a vein be distended with a larger than average amount of blood, a tourniquet should be applied. Natural rubber or latex tubing or a sphygmomanometer cuff serve as appropriate tourniquets.

It is best to apply a tourniquet 2 to 4 inches above the venipuncture site. It should be tightened only enough to distend the veins. Tourniquets tied too tightly can obstruct arterial flow and cause collapse of the veins. One method for ascertaining proper tourniquet fit is to check for presence of a pulse distal to the tourniquet. If the pulse is absent, the tourniquet is too tight.

When using a sphygmomanometer, the cuff should be inflated until the radial pulse ceases. Then release the cuff pressure to a point slightly below the patient's diastolic blood pressure (Plumer, 1975).

Should a sclerosed vein be utilized, it may be necessary to omit the use of a tourniquet, since pressure may cause the vein to become harder and tortuous (Plumer, 1975).

Methods for enhancing vein distention include heat application, light slapping of the skin over the vein, and milking of the veins by having the patient open and close his fist several times or manually stroking the part.

Heat application produces dilatation of the veins with a resulting increase in blood flow. Heat may be applied in the form of warm, moist compresses for 15 to 20 minutes or by soaking the part in a basin of warm water. It is important to note that heat application is far more effective when applied to the entire part than only to the injection site. The tissue response to heat is called reflex or reactive hyperemia (Newman, 1952).

Light slapping of the skin, fist-clenching, and stroking of the part produce a response known as mechanical reflex dilatation. The superficial veins and capillaries respond reflexively by relaxing the tone of the walls, allowing greater distention with blood. Too vigorous slapping, clenching, or stroking may produce an opposite effect just as emotional excitement, fear, or anxiety may reduce circulation to limbs (Newman, 1952; Adriani, 1962).

Should all else fail, the ischemic reactive hyperemia technique may be employed. This is accomplished by occluding arterial blood flow with a tourniquet. Once the tourniquet is released, maximum blood flow will follow. The scientific principle is that the blood vessels are responding to a previous ischemic state by rapidly dilating (Newman, 1952).

TAPE

One-half-inch adhesive, silk, or paper tape may be used to anchor the needle or cannulae to the skin. Water-repellant tape is preferred. The tape should be placed in such a manner as to prevent any to-or-fro movement of the device.

Criss-crossing of a strip of one-half-inch tape at the needle or cannula hub or wing taping are effective methods of securing the device. It is advisable to avoid placing tape over the venipuncture site, since the tape used is unsterile and having tape over the site makes it difficult to carry out IV site care.

Additional taping is necessary to secure the arm or hand board, to secure a loop of tubing, and to secure the site dressing. One-inch tape is used for this purpose.

Two to three strips of one-inch tape, backed with one-inch roller gauze, may be used for securing the arm or hand board to the patient.

Caution in taping is necessary in order to prevent nerve damage to the part. A rule is to apply the tape in such a manner as to immobilize the needle or cannula and at the same time allow the part to maintain a functional position.

ANTI-INFECTIVE AGENTS

The Center for Disease Control considers tincture of iodine as being the most effective agent for cleansing IV sites. Povidone iodine or 70% isopropyl alcohol are commonly used (Fig. 3-10). Controversy does exist regarding which anti-infective agent is most effective in killing and inhibiting the growth of microorganisms at the IV site.

Application of an antimicrobial ointment at the portal of entry after venipuncture, and every 24 hours thereafter for the duration of therapy, will considerably reduce the incidence of skin and systemic infection. Plain antibiotic ointments have been shown to be less effective than the combination ointments, particularly when plastic cannulae are used, since there is generally an overgrowth of fungus, especially *Candida albicans*, with these devices.

A portable rolling-type or bed-attachable standard may be selected. Patient condition, activity, and the type of therapy are factors to consider when selecting an intravenous standard.

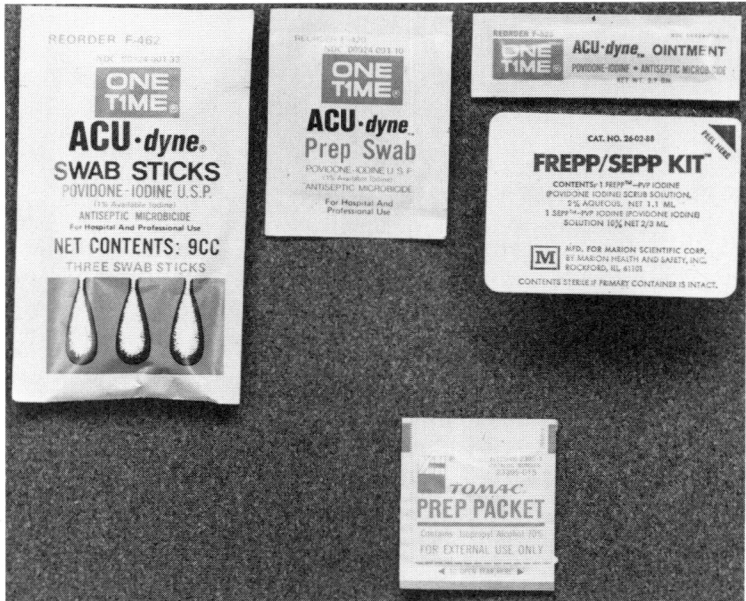

Fig. 3-10. Commonly used antiinfective agents. (Courtesy Alton Ochsner Medical Foundation, New Orleans.)

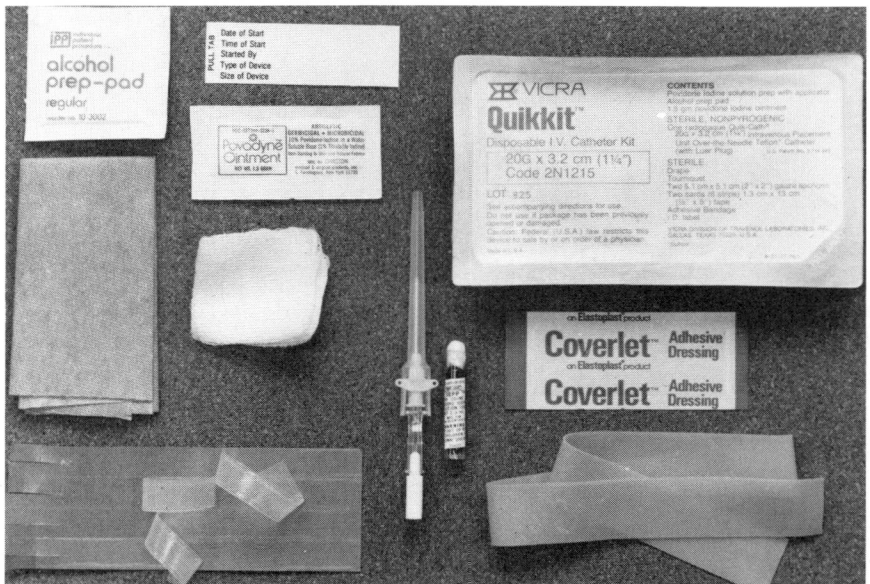

Fig. 3-11. Basic equipment for venipuncture. Infusion fluid not included. (Courtesy Alton Ochsner Medical Foundation, New Orleans.)

The infusion tubing drip chamber, when suspended approximately 3 feet from the site of injection, will achieve maximum flow rate due to the force of gravity. The greater the height, the greater the force of flow.

INFUSION PUMPS AND CONTROLLERS

Mechanical devices that serve to pump fluid into the patient and control rates of flow are sometimes attached to the infusion system.

Rates of flow are regulated through special pump or controller sensor devices.

Mechanical devices may fail, and therefore it is important for the nurse to monitor the patient and the pump or controller at frequent intervals.

Procedure

The following procedure delineates the essential steps and key points of venipuncture for the purpose of medication administration and starting a continuous and intermittent infusion.

There are certain parallels for each procedure. The appropriate needle or cannula, fluid, medication, tubing, filter, tourniquet, tape, anti-infective agent, IV standard, and sterile sponges must be gathered and placed on a cart or tray (Fig. 3-11).

Prior to starting, the patient should be psychologically and physically prepared. Principles for this preparation are discussed in a previous section of this chapter.

Essential steps	Key points
1. Obtain and adjust IV standard.	
2. Tear tape.	
3. Select IV site.	
4. Position and tie tourniquet and feel for vein.	
5. Release tourniquet and cleanse site with anti-infective agent.	Use friction and a circular motion, avoid contamination of site.
6. Retie tourniquet and feel for vein.	
7. Hold skin taut with thumb below injection site to anchor vein.	
8. Insert needle, bevel up, at 20-45 degree angle.	Insert directly over and into vein or along side of vein.
9. Lower hub of needle close to skin for thrust into vein.	A popping or snapping sound can be heard when the vein wall is penetrated; the needle should be on a straight course with the vein; backflow of blood into the puncturing device indicates satisfactory entry.

Essential steps	**Key points**
10. Enter vein slowly.	
11. Release tourniquet.	
12. Advance needle or cannula.	Thread with a slight uplifting motion to prevent puncturing inferior wall of vein.

13. Variations following threading are as follows:
    a. Infusions: Connect primed tubing and open tubing flow clamp and allow fluid to run at a fast rate to clear the tubing of blood. Observe for hematoma, pain, and infiltration. Discontinue the infusion should these things be observed and restart the infusion in another vein.
    b. Medication administration: Once backflow of blood appears in the syringe, remove the tourniquet and inject the medication in the time recommended. Observe the patient for expected action or reaction or both. Frequent checks for backflow of blood should be done by aspiration. Following injection of the medication, remove the needle, and apply pressure and a dry sterile dressing.
    c. Intermittent devices (heparin locks): Once backflow of blood appears, flush the set first with normal saline and second with a 1:9 heparin and normal saline solution (one part heparin, 1000 U/ml, and nine parts normal saline).
    d. Scalp vein or butterfly type needles: These should be connected to the primed intravenous tubing prior to venipuncture. A gentle squeeze on the tubing flash chamber will remove a small amount of fluid from the system, allowing space for blood backflow following venipuncture. Some nurses prefer to perform venipuncture prior to connecting the tubing. By following the recommended procedure, the fluid container can be attached to the IV standard, eliminating the need for placing the container below the injection site for ascertaining satisfactory entry into the vein.
    e. Over-the-needle cannulae: Once blood backflows into the flash chamber and threading is accomplished, which includes removal of its stylet, the primed IV tubing is connected.
    f. In-the-needle cannulae: Once blood backflow appears and threading is accomplished, the needle is removed and the primed IV tubing is connected. The fluid is allowed to run at a fast rate in order to clear the tubing of blood. Once cleared, the IV is regulated at the prescribed rate.

14. Tape needle or cannula.	Check extremity for circulation.
15. Apply antimicrobial ointment to venipuncture site.	
16. Apply 2 × 2 inch sterile dressing.	Label with date, time, and nurses name.
17. Apply arm or hand board.	Should IV be in naturally splinted area, this step may be omitted.
18. Loop and tape 3 to 6 inch portion of tubing.	Shorter loops may cause tubing to kink.

19. Review movement restrictions with patient.
20. Assist patient to allowed position of comfort.
21. Adjust flow rate.
22. Recheck flow rate, possibility of infiltration, and other complications every 30 to 60 minutes.
23. Dispose of used equipment.
24. Discontinue when indicated.
25. Record all pertinent information.

GENERAL INFORMATION

Complications such as pain, infiltration, and hematoma necessitates removal and restart at another site. Other complications are to be reported to the physician.

Solutions and tubings are to be changed each 24 hours.

IV sites should be rotated each 48 to 72 hours in order to assure maximum infection control. This, however, may not always be practical, since patient conditions and availability of veins vary.

Pressure on the injection site following removal of a needle or cannula should be maintained for 3 to 5 minutes or until bleeding stops. Following application of pressure, a sterile, dry dressing should be applied and maintained for approximately 24 hours.

The recorded information should include the amount and type of solution used, the type of needle and size, the site of venipuncture, medications and dosages added and by whom, and the rate of flow in milliliters per hour, since rates of flow in drops per minute are misleading because drop factors vary from tubing to tubing.

Pertinent observations such as anxiety and untoward reactions should be included in the record.

Sign all notes with first initial, surname, and title.

FACTORS AFFECTING FLOW RATE

In order to ensure therapeutic effectiveness of substances infusing into the patient's circulatory system, maintenance of a constant, even flow is necessary.

There are several factors that may alter prescribed and set flow rates, including venous pressure, vein spasms, development of phlebitis and thrombi, viscosity and specific gravity of the fluid, amount of fluid remaining in container, height of fluid container, tubing occlusion, use of filters, medication additions, needle or cannula size, needle or cannula position, needle and cannula occlusion, and infiltration.

Specific information about each of these factors as they relate to flow rates are to be considered.

Venous pressure

Normal venous pressure ranges from 5 to 14 cm of water. The infusion tubing drip chamber must be of sufficient height to overcome this pressure. A height of approximately 0.9 m (3 ft) above the injection site is considered adequate.

Should the patient be in a state of hypovolemia, venous pressure decreases and flow rates of fluids increase.

Vein spasms

This is a local myogenic spasm caused by trauma or damage to a blood vessel (Guyton, 1976). Irritating fluids and medications or chilled fluids and medications can set off a reflex action that sets the vein into spasms. Remedies for vein spasms include administration of medications only after adequate dilution, utilization of large veins and relatively small needles or cannulae when irritating fluids are used, and administering fluids and medications that are at room temperature.

Development of phlebitis and thrombi

As phlebitis and thrombi develop, the initial decrease in flow rate is due to spasm. As clots form and platelets disintegrate, a substance called serotonin is released, and in turn is believed to cause the smooth muscle to contract still more, intensifying the local contraction (Guyton, 1976).

Viscosity and specific gravity of fluid

Fluids such as those containing high concentrations of dextrose and blood tend to flow at slower rates. Height adjustment, utilization of needles and cannulae with larger than average lumen, and utilization of pumps may be required in order to deliver these substances at the prescribed rate.

Amount of fluid remaining in container

Since the weight of the remaining fluid is ever decreasing, the rate of flow may be ever decreasing.

Height of fluid container

The fluid container must be of sufficient height from the injection site to facilitate movement of the fluid from container through the tubing and into the patient. The tubing drip chamber, when suspended approximately 0.9 m (3 ft) from the injection site will, under the force of gravity, achieve maximum flow rate. The greater the height, the greater the force of flow.

Tubing occlusion

Most tubes have "memories" and therefore tend to compress while warm and remain compressed as temperatures cool. Studies reveal that flow rates change at 15-, 30-, 45-, and 60-minute intervals. As time sequences increase, rates of flow decrease. This is a major reason why it is necessary that flow rates be checked every 30 to 60 minutes.

Tubing occlusion may occur through kinking. The patient may be lying on a tube, creating a kink, or the tubing may have been improperly taped.

Tubing occlusion occurs when air vents clog. This may be due to inadequate placement of a needle that serves as a vent or when vents are too small to accommodate the viscosity of the fluid being infused. Vents should be checked for proper functioning prior to discontinuing an infusion that is dripping sluggishly or has stopped.

Use of filters

As in-line filters collect particulate matter and other wastes they become sluggish and eventually clog. It is recommended that filters be changed according to product information recommendations, and more frequently if indicated.

Medication additions

Crystallization of medications may occur within the infusion system because of incompatibilities or inadequate dilution. This results in flow rate changes. Medications incompletely dissolved may trap in the in-line filter and occlude the system.

Needle or cannula size

The smaller the needle or cannula lumen, the slower the fluid will flow. The rate of flow of any given solution decreases in proportion to the viscosity of the fluid while the flow of fluid varies inversely with the length of the needle shaft. A longer needle, while all other conditions are equal, may actually reduce the rate of flow of a given solution (Adriani, 1962).

Needle and cannula position

Should the bevel of the needle or cannula adhere to the wall of a vein, the flow of fluid may be disrupted. Repositioning of the needle or cannula by propping it or turning it and immobilization of the part may remedy this problem.

Needle and cannula occlusion

The causative factors for needle and cannula occlusion may be thrombi formation within the lumen or a kink in the cannula.

The onset of thrombi formation may be gradual due to a gradual buildup of blood cells and platelets within the lumen, or the onset may be sudden following occlusion of the flow of fluid from any point within the system or when the fluid container is of inadequate height, causing a backflow of blood into the needle, cannula, or tubing.

Infiltration

Should a needle or cannula slip out of a vein or inadvertently puncture the superior or inferior wall of a vein, the fluid or medication will
extravasate into the surrounding tissue. As the fluid or medication infiltrates the surrounding tissue, edema ensues. Extravasation many
times continues until such time as the tissue space is filled to capacity.
At this point the flow will cease.

VENOUS CUTDOWNS (VENISECTION)

Conditions requiring venous cutdowns include absence of superficial veins due to obesity and other conditions such as a need for prolonged therapy and cardiac arrest when venous collapse is present.

An incision is made at the probable vein location. The vein is iso-

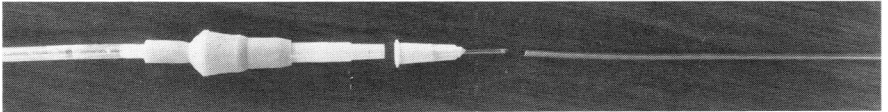

Fig. 3-12. Inlying type catheter for use with venous cutdowns (venisection).
(Courtesy Alton Ochsner Medical Foundation, New Orleans.)

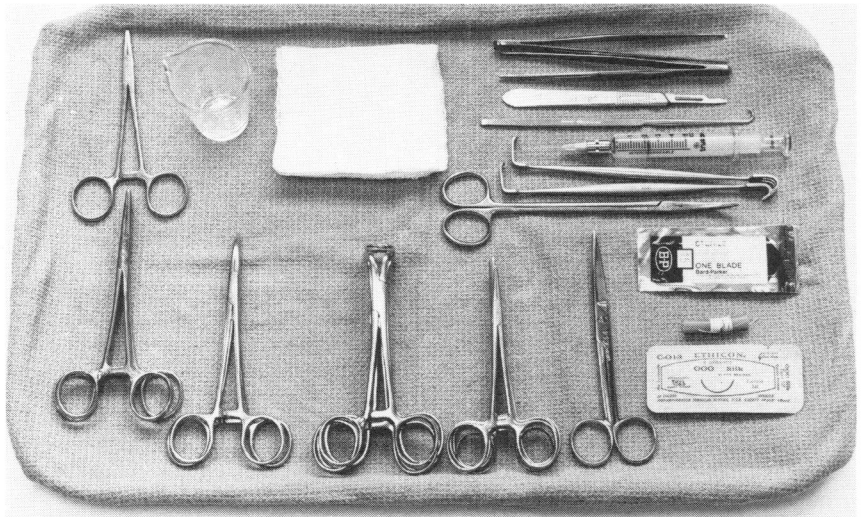

Fig. 3-13. Equipment needed for performing a venous cutdown (venisection).
(Courtesy Alton Ochsner Medical Foundation, New Orleans.)

lated and incised, and a plastic inlying type catheter is inserted and threaded into the vein (Figs. 3-12 and 3-13). Once the infusion is established, the catheter is sutured in place and the skin incision is sutured (Plumer, 1975).

HYPODERMOCLYSIS

Hypodermoclysis is the subcutaneous administration of sterile injectable fluids. This therapy may be useful for the obese, elderly, and pediatric patient, since superficial veins in these patients may not be readily accessible.

Sites of administration include the lateral thigh, abdomen, and subscapular areas. Caution should be exercised during puncture so that blood vessels are avoided. In the case of the subscapular site, the pleura should be avoided.

Only those fluids that resemble the tonicity of the extracellular fluid should be used. Examples of the fluids are 0.9% saline, 0.45% saline with 2.5% dextrose, Ringer's solution, half-strength Ringer's solution with 2.5% dextrose, lactated Ringer's solution, half-strength lactated Ringer's solution with 2.5% dextrose, and Darrow's solution.

The appropriate fluid is connected to a "Y" type infusion tubing specifically designed for hypodermoclysis. This tubing is a double tubing and has an attachment for two needles. Both needles are generally inserted at two separate sites at a 25- to 30-degree angle with bevel down. The skin is prepared in the usual manner and the puncture is made. The needles are secured in place with tape, and a sterile dressing with a suitable antimicrobial ointment is applied over the injection site.

The fluid may be administered from both sites simultaneously or sequentially at 1- to 2-hour intervals.

Absorption of the fluid is enhanced by the addition of the enzyme hyaluronidase (Wydase) to the fluid container or by injecting it at the clysis site.

The rate of flow is most often determined by the rate of fluid absorption. Edema at the injection site is an indication of rate of absorption.

Strict aseptic procedures should be adhered to, since edematous injection sites are susceptible to infection. (Brunner and Suddarth, 1975; Plumer, 1975).

References

Adriani, J.: Venipuncture, Am. J. Nurs. **62:**3, 1962.
Alton Ochsner Medical Foundation, Hospital Division, Department of Nursing Service, Staff Development Procedure Manual, New Orleans, 1977, The Foundation.
Anthony, C. A., and Thibodeau, G. A.: Textbook of anatomy and physiology, ed. 10, St. Louis, 1979, The C. V. Mosby Co.

Brunner, L., and Suddarth, D.: Textbook of Medical-Surgical Nursing, ed. 3, Philadelphia, 1975, J. B. Lippincott Co.

Center for Disease Control: Recommendations for the prevention of IV associated infections, Atlanta, 1973, Bacterial Diseases Branch, Bureau of Epidemiology.

Guyton, A.: Textbook of medical physiology, ed. 5, Philadelphia, 1976, W. B. Saunders Co.

IV sets and why IV therapy, Nursing 72, Oct. 1972.

Newman, E.: Technic of venipuncture and intravenous injection, Am. J. Nurs. **52:**4, 1952.

Plumer, A.: Principles and practice of intravenous therapy, ed. 2, Boston, 1975, Little, Brown & Co.

Thomas, C., editor: Taber's cyclopedic medical dictionary, ed. 13, Philadelphia, 1977, F. A. Davis Co.

Chapter 4

Intravenous medications

The nurse's responsibilities regarding administration of medications by way of the intravenous route are not too different from those required during administration of medications by other means. Since the dangers involved in administering medications by this route are great, special emphasis must be placed in most areas of the nurse's responsibility.

It is intended that the information in this chapter will help to increase the nurse's knowledge of the rationale underlying the intravenous drug therapy, assist the nurse in learning to use this knowledge clinically to recognize both therapeutic and deleterious effects of drug therapy, and assist the nurse in identifying appropriate nursing action (Del Bueno et al., 1971).

GENERAL INFORMATION AND RESPONSIBILITIES

Numerous medications are unstable in the presence of gastric juices. Some medications, because of their large molecular size, are not absorbed by the gastrointestinal route. Some medications, because of their irritating properties, cause pain and trauma when administered subcutaneously or intramuscularly.

The intravenous route provides for rapid absorption and instantaneous action of medications; continuous administration and control over the rate of administration of medications; a method of administering medications to patients who cannot tolerate fluids and medications by the gastrointestinal route; and immediate termination of the therapy should sensitivity occur.

The nurse must be knowledgeable regarding the drug to be administered. A review of each drug prior to its administration is vital. Information concerning drugs administered during emergencies should be imprinted in the mind of the nurse, since when an emergency arises, there may be little time to review the reference material. Most agencies

55

have a list of drugs commonly used during emergencies. Independent study is most often indicated.

The following categories of information are to be reviewed prior to the administration of intravenous medications: drug classification; actions, indications, and uses (cause and effect); side effects, precautions, and contraindications; incompatibilities; antidotes; dosage; dilution; rate of administration; onset of action, rate of absorption, and circulation time; and nursing points.

The following discussion includes the aforementioned categories and those aspects of drug information that require special consideration in terms of intravenous therapy.

Drug classification

Drugs possessing similarities in chemical structure and biologic activity are categorized into families or classes.

General information concerning each class of drugs and specific information concerning each drug within the class is to be reviewed prior to intravenous administration.

The example used in this text is drugs used to treat cardiac arrhythmias.

Drugs classified as antiarrhythmics, although belonging to several different chemical groups, exert specific action on the electrical activity of cardiac muscle cells. The result is a decrease in number and frequency of ectopic heart beats or a return of normal cardiac rhythm.

During administration of antiarrhythmics the patient's electrocardiogram is to be continuously monitored and the medication is to be discontinued when the arrhythmia is corrected or when the patient's cardiac condition is stable (Rodman and Smith, 1974).

Consider that the following drugs are approved to be administered by way of the intravenous route because of the antiarrhythmic effect: lidocaine hydrochloride, procainamide hydrochloride, quinidine gluconate injection, phenytoin sodium, and propranolol hydrochloride. Specific information as it relates to each of these drugs is as follows:

1. Lidocaine hydrochloride—keep a bolus dose, 100 mg in 5 ml, available at all times for emergency use in myocardial infarction; convulsions may occur.
2. Procainamide or quinidine—cross-sensitivity and potentiation may occur.
3. Procainamide hydrochloride—protect from light and store in refrigerator; discard if solution is darker than light amber; use care with digitalis, lidocaine, and quinidine, since lower doses of both drugs may be required.
4. Quinidine gluconate—too rapid administration may cause a

marked decrease in arterial pressure; potentiated by neuromuscular blocking antibiotics, anticholinergics, thiazide diuretics, antihypertensive agents, muscle relaxants, anticoagulants, and others; cardiac arrhythmias may occur.

5. Phenytoin sodium—determine absolute patency of vein; avoid extravasation, very alkaline; follow each injection with sterile normal saline to reduce local venous irritation; incompatible with many drugs and will precipitate if pH is altered.

6. Propranolol hydrochloride—central venous pressure monitoring is mandatory during intravenous administration; should be discontinued 48 hours prior to major surgery, since beta blockade interferes with cardiac response to reflex stimuli (Gahart, 1977).

Actions, indications, and uses (cause and effect)

A review of drug actions, indications, and uses (cause and effect) provides information related to how the drug works, what action it has within the body, diseases or conditions for which it is recommended, and what effect may be anticipated.

There is recorded evidence indicating errors in judgment on the part of nurses who have failed to realize cause and effect. As an example, consider a nurse caring for a patient admitted into a hospital with a problem related to muscle spasm in the lumbar region of his back. The physician ordered the patient to receive diazepam 5 mg every 4 hours continuously. The nurse on duty at the time of the incident assessed that the patient was resting comfortably and therefore omitted two doses of the diazepam. During the 8 hours that the diazepam was omitted, the nurse administered codeine, since the patient complained of "spasms in his low back." It is obvious that the nurse did not realize the cause and effect, for if she had, she would have administered diazepam as ordered. The indications and uses for diazepam include treatment of muscle spasms, stress, convulsions, cardioversion, alcohol withdrawal, and preoperative sedation. Had the diazepam been administered, the patient possibly would not have required codeine.

Side effects, precautions, and contraindications

Drug side effects are those effects that occur in addition to those for which the drug was intended. Side effects may be helpful, harmful, or innocuous. Harmful side effects are many times referred to as untoward effects (Rodman and Smith, 1974). Precautions are measures taken to guard against untoward effects. Contraindications dictate that certain medications may be harmful if administered in the presence of certain conditions or other medications.

Included in the review of specific information related to side effects, precautions, and contraindications are drug allergies; failing or failed systems of the body; patient conditions such as age, weight, and states of debilitation; drugs the patient is receiving that may potentiate, inhibit, synergize or antagonize; monitoring of vital signs, electrocardiogram, and the like; need for presence of the physician during administration; loss of drug potency following reconstitution or exposure to light; avoidance of prolonged use; caution when used in certain situations such as pregnancy; hematologic and chemical values; dangers of vein irritation; and warnings regarding habituation and addiction.

Incompatibilities

The *American Heritage Dictionary* (1973) defines incompatible as "not compatible; inharmonious; antagonistic"; and compatible as "capable of living or performing in harmonious combination with others; capable or orderly, efficient integration and operation with other elements in the system."

Incompatibility of medications and solutions means that the medications and solutions do not conform or adapt to each other because they are not similar in their chemical nature.

When medications and solutions incompatible with each other are mixed together, the chemical reactions that occur may be serious. Either may be rendered lethal or partially to totally ineffective.

There are four definite chemical reactions that may occur. Hydrolysis, where there is a chemical splitting of a compound of salt by water, produces either a strong acid and a weak base or a weak acid and a strong base. The opposite of hydrolysis is neutralization. Since the pH of a substance determines acidity or alkalinity of the substance, one can see how an incompatibility can occur through hydrolysis.

Reduction, the second reaction, occurs when one substance gains electrons from the other, causing the valence of the substance to decrease, thereby decreasing its combining power.

Oxidation, the third reaction, occurs when one substance loses electrons to the other, causing the valence of the substance to increase. This process occurs while reduction is taking place. Certain antioxidants (preservatives) are added to substances to prevent oxidation.

Double decomposition, the fourth reaction, is a chemical change in which the molecules of two interacting compounds exchange a portion of their constituents.

Incompatibilities may be visible or invisible. That is to say, some are seen by the naked eye and some are not.

Visible incompatibilities are generally easily detected. On the other hand, invisible incompatibilities are of greater concern, since recognition by inspection is virtually impossible. It is because of this that concern regarding pH of all medications and solutions is vital.

Drastic changes in pH are produced when strong acids and weak bases are mixed. This alters the stability of the substance.

When substances that are insoluble in solution are mixed, a precipitation occurs. Solubility may vary with the pH (Plumer, 1975).

pH, or the stability of a medication or solution, can be altered by the pH of either the medication or solution that is being mixed, the addition of a second or third medication, the buffering agent within the medication, the preservative within the diluent being used to reconstitute the medication, the concentration of medication in solution, the time lapse between reconstitution of a medication and its addition to a solution, the order in which medications are added to the solution, light, and temperature.

Incompatibilities may be classified as therapeutic, physical, chemical, and physiologic (Plumer, 1975). Therapeutic incompatibilities result when incompatible medications are either given at the same time or sequentially. Physical incompatibilities produced by physical or chemical reactions cause visible or invisible changes to occur. Examples include color changes, precipitation, and the formation of gas. Chemical incompatibilities produce reactions that are invisible. This type of reaction may go undetected, and therefore awareness that this type of incompatibility can occur is vital. Physiologic incompatibilities occur when one or more substances, mixed in solution, produce an antagonistic effect to one of the substances.

Most large institutions of health care have admixture services that are usually components of the pharmacy department. In addition to having the capability of admixing intravenous medications in a clean air environment (laminar flow), the mixer is trained to be acutely aware of all potential incompatibilities. Current charts and other reference material on the subject of incompatibilities are also available.

In smaller institutions the role of admixer is usually taken by the nurse. With this in mind it is recommended that awareness of the potentially dangerous effects of administering medications and solutions that are incompatible be of paramount importance. Current charts and other reference materials related to incompatibilities should be made available (Fig. 4-1).

Since incompatibilities are continuously being discovered, it is advisable to review all current literature specific to the medication to be administered. Should there be no available information on the patient care unit, it is advisable to consult the agency's pharmacist.

Some specific points are to never mix two or more drugs in the same

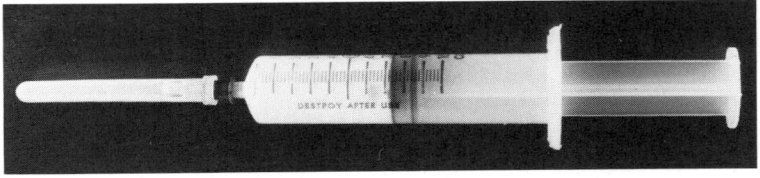

Fig. 4-1. Milky-white precipitate in syringe—a visible incompatibility. (Courtesy Alton Ochsner Medical Foundation, New Orleans.)

syringe prior to administration. Since incompatibility may be determined by the order in which the medications are admixed, drugs should be admixed in correct sequence.

All warnings regarding utilization of specific diluents and recommendations concerning administration of drugs in concentrated or diluted form should be heeded.

Medications should be protected from light and stored in refrigerators as indicated.

Antidotes

Antidotes may consist of medications and treatments used to counteract untoward effects of intravenous medications.

Some antidotes act to antagonize or neutralize the toxic agent, while others provide supportive therapy.

The nurse should anticipate which medication or treatment will be required, and all necessary equipment should be available for use.

A physician's order is required for the administration of all antidotes. Conditions that necessitate the use of antidotes are many times considered crisis periods. The presence of the physician is recommended during the acute phase.

Other measures used during this period include cardiopulmonary resuscitation, artificial ventilation, and monitoring of vital signs and cardiac rhythm. It is recommended that all nurses performing the function of administering drugs by the intravenous route be trained in cardiopulmonary resuscitation (CPR). CPR can be initiated without an order from the physician.

Should untoward effects occur, the pernicious medication is to be discontinued and the physician notified. The crisis is dealt with through collaboration with the physician and other members of the health care team.

Crisis is many times prevented by administering only that amount of medication that the patient can tolerate. This is especially related to the administration of tranquilizers, narcotics, barbiturates, and sedatives.

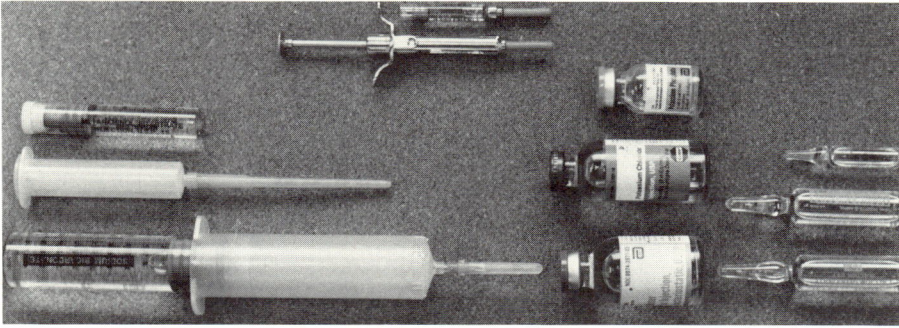

Fig. 4-2. Medications and diluents. (Courtesy Alton Ochsner Medical Foundation, New Orleans.)

Dosage

The usual dosage of a medication is indicative of that dose of a drug that has been established as therapeutically effective when used in most circumstances.

The dosage range of a drug is the minimum and maximum amounts of a drug that will provide therapeutic effectiveness.

The maintenance dosage of a drug is that amount of a drug that will, when administered on a regular schedule, maintain therapeutic effectiveness.

In reviewing specific points related to dosages of intravenous medications, it is necessary that recommended dosages be administered. In life-threatening situations, maximum recommended daily dosages are sometimes exceeded. The patient's condition and the possible effectiveness of some other agent should be considered before attempts are made to exceed what is proven to be safe and effective.

Dilution

Medications intended for intravenous administration are available in aqueous and nonaqueous solutions, lyophilized powders requiring reconstitution with aqueous diluents, and lyophilized powders requiring reconstitution with special diluents (Francke, 1973) (Fig. 4-2).

Medications improperly reconstituted may not obtain the desired chemical composition. Methods for reconstituting the medication, the type of diluent to use, and the amount of fluid into which the medication is to be added are to be reviewed and followed.

Certain diluents may contain preservatives and, as such, may be incompatible with the drug to be administered. When underdiluted or overdiluted, the effects of some drugs may be altered. In addition, serious vein irritation may occur.

Sound infection control practice incorporates the utilization of new, unopened vials and ampules of diluent, since previously used containers may have been contaminated with microorganisms or incompatible substances.

Multiple-dose vials of drugs intended for intravenous administration should be labeled with the date and time of reconstitution. Include the dose contained in each milliliter, the name of the nurse reconstituting the drug, and the expiration date. Refrigerate or protect from heat and light as indicated by the product information.

Rate of administration

Rates of administration vary according to the method used, that is to say, drugs diluted in a large quantity of fluid such as a continuous infusion; drugs diluted in a moderate quantity of fluid such as a piggyback; and drugs diluted in a small quantity of fluid such as an intravenous push medication.

Consideration is given to the site of administration, such as peripheral lines where a drug such as glucose could cause irritation and sclerosis of the vein, and central venous administration where the drug could conceivably have a direct irritating effect on the heart muscle.

Medications are to be timed as they are administered. If administered too fast or too slow, the effects could be altered. As an example, medications administered in high concentrations can produce speed shock. This is a systemic reaction when a substance foreign to the body is rapidly introduced into the circulation. The rapid injection of a drug permits its concentration in the plasma to reach toxic proportions, flooding the organs rich in blood. The results are syncope, shock, and cardiac arrest (Plumer, 1975).

Onset of action, rate of absorption, and circulation time

Onset of action is that time following injection that drug action occurs. Absorption of a drug is the movement of a drug molecule from the site of injection to the circulating fluids. In intravenous administration of medications the onset of action and rate of absorption is instantaneous.

Normal circulation time ranges from 18 to 24 seconds. This time is altered by circulatory conditions.

Nursing points

Nursing points serve to delineate the nurse's overall responsibility regarding intravenous medication administration. This includes the nurse's preparation prior to administration and observations before, during, and after administration.

Accept only those physician orders that contain all components. That is, drug name, dosage and strength, route or method (such as continuous infusion, IV piggyback, or IV push), and frequency of administration. Orders reading IV warrant clarification, since IV does not denote the method of administration.

Review the drug literature prior to administration. Be familiar with all possible and probable complications. Know what to do in the event of a crisis. Should adverse effects occur, discontinue the medication and notify the physician. Be aware of both independent and dependent actions required to keep the entire process a safe one.

Drugs intended for IV piggyback or IV push administration are not to be mixed; instead administer one drug at a time. Drugs mixed in a continuous infusion should be done only after careful consideration and consultation with incompatability lists and the agency's pharmacist.

Stop or discontinue the medication once the effectiveness is reached. Slurred speech in the case of barbiturates is a prime indicator of onset of toxicity. Sound judgment and common sense is important.

Be aware of the dangers of mechanical and chemical irritation, sloughing, and phlebitis.

If there is a question regarding a dose that has been calculated, consult with another registered nurse. Be mindful of the old but forever true adage, "when in doubt, don't."

Use in-line, syringe, or needle type filters in order to remove bacteria, particulate matter, and air from the system being used.

Dilute the medication in an even amount of solution in order to afford accuracy in delivery of the medication. That is to say, when a medication is diluted in an even amount of fluid, such as 10 mg of medication in 10 ml of fluid, there is exactly 1 mg in each 1 ml, ¾ mg in ¾ ml, ½ mg in ½ ml, ¼ mg in ¼ ml, and so on. As the medication is being administered, the exact amount administered can be determined at a glance.

Know the patient's diagnosis and his or her current and past health status. Keep all previously described information regarding reactions to drugs in mind. Assessment of the patient's condition and probable response is vital.

Use the laminar flow hood when possible for admixing continuous infusions and piggyback medications. It is not always possible to prepare IV push medications under a laminar flow hood; however, the advantages regarding infection control can be imagined.

Several techniques may help reduce vein irritation. For IV push administration, use the smallest gauge needle possible. The small needle serves as a safety valve in that the push, even with forceful pressure, will be slower than with a larger gauge needle, thus allowing for adequate dilution of the drug as the blood flow through the veins. Use hepa-

rinized saline following a 50 to 100 ml dose of antibiotic to aid in preventing thrombi formation and vein irritation at the injection site. This
is specific to intermittent infusion sets. Use intermittent infusions such
as piggybacks rather than a continuous infusion. This allows the vein
to rest between doses. Ten to 25 mg of hydrocortisone can be added to
the primary IV solution to aid in reducing inflammation at the site of
injection with no significant systemic effect. When possible, use normal
saline as the intravenous fluid or diluent during medication therapy.
Normal saline has a more neutral pH than 5% dextrose in water or sterile water for injection and is therefore less irritating. Attempt to avoid
using bacteriostatic water with benzyl alcohol as a preservative. The
alcohol is irritating to the vein if given in an undiluted solution. Use
at least 50 to 100 ml of diluent with all antibiotics. This aids in reducing the concentration of the medication and therefore is less irritating. The use of solutions neutralized with sodium bicarbonate is advisable, since the pH values of the solutions are near normal. For IV
therapy extending beyond 72 hours, it is recommended that injection
sites be rotated.

METHODS OF ADMINISTRATION

Medications are administered intravenously by way of continuous
and intermittent infusions through peripheral and central veins.

With continuous infusions the medication is diluted in a relatively
large amount of fluid (low concentration of medication). The amount
of fluid may vary from 250 ml to 500 to 1000 ml, and the solution is
delivered over a 2- to 24-hour period.

Intermittent infusions of medications are delivered through piggybacks in which the medication is diluted in a relatively moderate
amount of fluid, usually 10 to 150 ml, an average being 50 to 100 ml
administered over a 5-minute to 2-hour period (moderate concentration
of medication).

Intermittent infusions of medications are also delivered by IV push
in which the medication is diluted in a relatively small amount of fluid,
usually 0.25 to 50 ml and administered over a 5-second to 5-minute
period (high concentration of medicine).

Medications are also administered by IV push by direct venipuncture.

There are situations where the administration time for IV push may
be extended to 10 to 15 minutes. Such situations include the patient's
condition, the time available, drug, effect desired, and an order from
the physician.

Since highly concentrated medications sometimes have a direct irritating effect on the endocardium, extreme caution is necessary when medications are administered by way of central lines.

The pharmacist is charged with the responsibility of compounding and dispensing medications. Admixture services instituted by many health care agencies provide for preparation of all intravenous fluids and their additives by pharmacists. Advantages of this service include the pharmacist's utilization of the laminar flow hood and availability of multiple resource materials.

EQUIPMENT

Equipment used in administering medications by the intravenous route includes syringes, needles, bags and bottles, primary and secondary tubings, microdrop tubings, filters, and, in some cases, pumps and controllers.

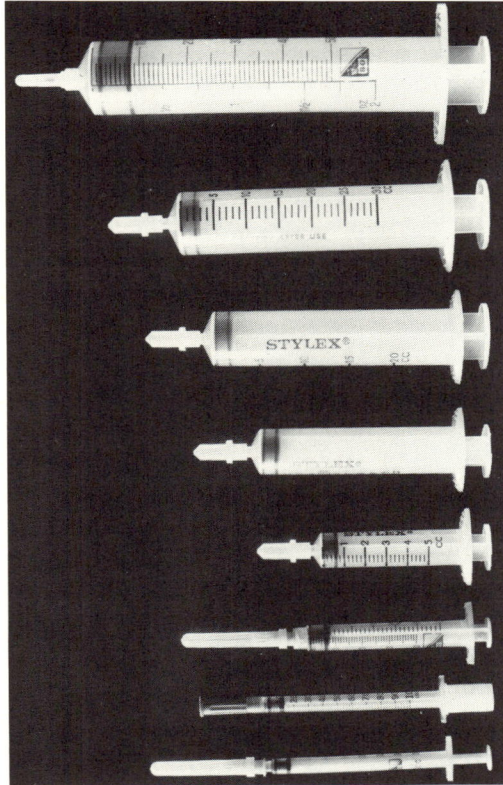

Fig. 4-3. Syringes commonly used to administer intravenous medications. (Courtesy Alton Ochsner Medical Foundation, New Orleans.)

Syringes

The syringes used to administer intravenous medications are insulin, tuberculin, and either catheter-tip or luer-lock syringes of the 2, 3, 5, 10, 20, 30, and 50 ml size. The choice of syringe is determined by the medication to be administered and the volume of the solution (Fig. 4-3).

Needles

The needles commonly used are 18, 19, 20, 21, 22, 23, and 25 gauge (Fig. 4-4).

Needle selection depends on its purpose. As examples, an 18-gauge needle is appropriate for drawing diluents from vials or ampules, since the size of the lumen facilitates rapid withdrawal; however, a needle of this size may capture a bore of rubber from the vial, which may be introduced into the final solution to be administered to the patient. Such a problem is avoided when solutions are filtered.

In contrast, a 23- or 25-gauge needle may slow the process of withdrawal. A slower infusion rate, which is frequently desirable, can be anticipated with smaller gauge needles.

Bags and bottles

Bag or bottle solution containers are used to administer intravenous medications.

Some authorities feel that bags are hazardous in that particles of plastic may be introduced into the patient; portions of the medication added may cling to the walls of the bag and drip out as the bag is emp-

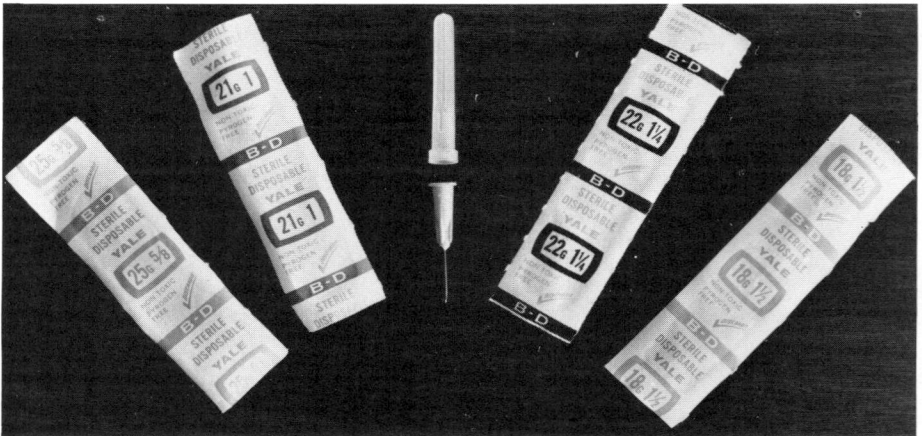

Fig. 4-4. Some needles commonly used to prepare and administer intravenous medications. (Courtesy Alton Ochsner Medical Foundation, New Orleans.)

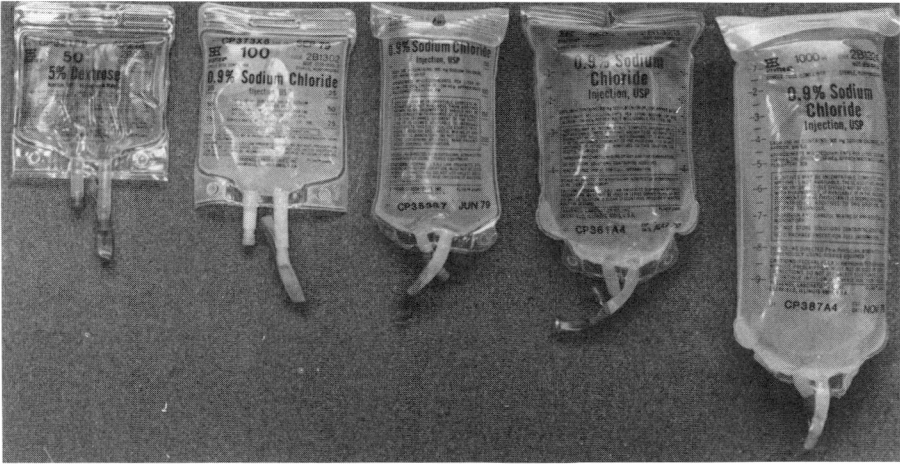

Fig. 4-5. IV bags. (Courtesy Alton Ochsner Medical Foundation, New Orleans.)

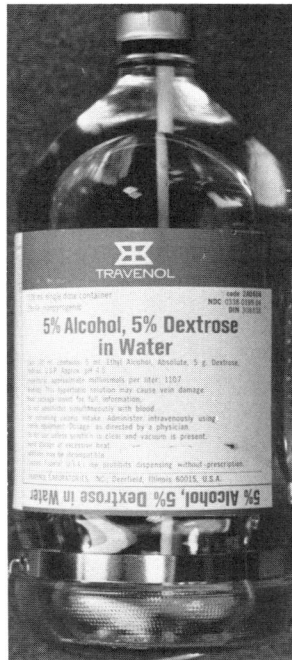

Fig. 4-6. IV bottle. (Courtesy Alton Ochsner Medical Foundation, New Orleans.)

tying, causing the patient to receive a bolus of medication; and plastic absorbs portions of the medication and therefore the patient does not reap full benefit from the prescribed dose (Fig. 4-5).

The major objections to using bottles are that glass particles may be administered to the patient, and since bottles require venting, the patient is predisposed to air embolism (Fig. 4-6).

In considering bags versus bottles, bags provide a closed system and therefore are preferred in terms of infection control.

The introduction of plastic or glass particles and air into the patient is minimized when in-line filters are utilized.

Primary and secondary tubings

The primary tubing is that which is connected to the continuous infusion. The secondary tubing is that which is superimposed or piggy-backed into the primary line by way of the rubber flash chamber or by way of a tubing side arm.

Repeated sticks into rubber reseal injection sites can cause leaking at the site, particularly when needles of gauges larger than 22 are used. Since most agencies practice the Center for Disease Control recommendation of changing tubings each 24 hours, this problem has been, to a large extent, eliminated.

Advances in intravenous piggyback administration of medications includes the use of tubings with check valves. Check valves prevent backflow of fluid and medication from or equidistant to the injection site by utilizing the principle of hydrostatic pressure. That is to say, when the primary IV bag is lowered below the smaller secondary bag, hydrostatic pressure causes the check valve within the primary tubing to lift, causing the primary tubing to temporarily shut off, and allowing the secondary set to flow. Once the secondary set empties, the check valve from the primary set will lower, allowing the primary set to flow.

Microdrop tubings

Microdrop tubings use the 60 drops/ml factor. Microdrop tubings are used for keep-open infusions and for administration of fluid and medication at 50 ml/hour or less.

Microdrop tubings are of the straight tubing and burette types. A problem related to the burette type tubing is that close observation is required since, once the burette empties, additional fluid will have to be added in order that patency of the infusion is maintained. Microdrop sets of the burette type pose no great problem when used in intensive care areas or large wards where continuous observation is possible (Fig. 4-7).

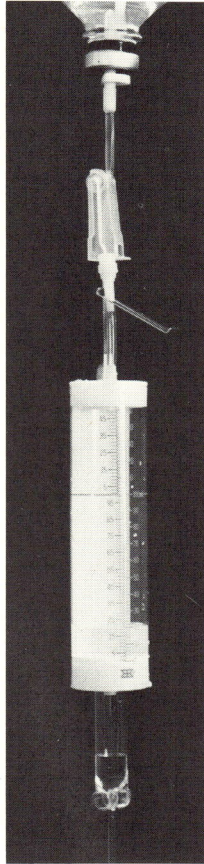

Fig. 4-7. Burette type microdrop tubing commonly used for IV piggyback administration of medications. (Courtesy Alton Ochsner Medical Foundation, New Orleans.)

Filters

In-line and final filters, when properly wetted, remove particulate matter, air, and some or all bacteria from the solution being administered.

Infusion pumps and controllers

Infusion pumps and controllers are electrical or battery-operated devices that, when connected to the IV tubing, control or pump the fluid and medication being administered to the patient in a specified period of time.

Nursing time in monitoring flow rates can be drastically reduced, and barring any mechanical or electrical failure, pumps and controllers assure that the patient will receive a given amount of fluid or medication in a given period of time. Although the advantages of using these devices far outweigh the disadvantages, it is the wise nurse who remembers to nurse the patient and not the machine.

PROCEDURES

The procedures for administering intravenous medications are continuous infusion, intravenous push (basic, by venipuncture, and by the various needles and cannulae during compatible and incompatible situations), and intravenous piggyback.

Included in this section are the purpose of each procedure, essential steps, and key points.

Prior to administration, the patient should be physically and psychologically prepared. Principles for this preparation are discussed in a previous chapter.

Continuous infusion method

The purpose of the continuous infusion method is to administer one or more medications to a patient in a relatively long period of time, usually over a 2- to 24-hour period. Medications administered by this method are first diluted in a relatively large amount of fluid, usually 250, 500, or 1000 ml.

Essential steps	Key points
1. Admix medication(s) with IV fluid.	Verify compability; use laminar flow hood if available.
2. Label container with patient's name, room number, container number, medication(s) added, dosage, rate of administration in ml/hour, admixer's name and title, time prepared, and expiration date.	
3. Water clock or time tape container.	
4. Connect and prime appropriate tubing and filter.	
5. Identify patient.	
6. Start infusion.	See procedure in Chapter 3.
7. Adjust flow rate as prescribed.	
8. Observe every 30 to 60 minutes.	
9. Add subsequent containers as prescribed.	
10. Discontinue when completed.	
11. Record all pertinent information (Fig. 4-8).	

Intravenous push method

The purpose of the intravenous push method is to administer one or more medications to a patient in a relatively short period of time,

NURSES' NOTES

Date	Time			Signature
6-1-78	8 AM	#1) 1000 ml DSW c̄	Started per I.V. in	
		20 mEq KCl	Ⓛ Ant. forearm c̄	
			#21 gauge S.V.	
			needle	
		Infusing	at 125 ml/h	B. Brown, RN
	4 PM	Infusion	Completed and dc'd	S. Smith, RN

Fig. 4-8. Nurses' notes recording of continuous infusion.

usually 5 seconds to 5 minutes. This method allows for administration of medications only following reconstitution or dilution or both with 0.25 to 50 ml of an appropriate diluent. Literature on each drug, found in package inserts and reference books, are appropriate guides for determining the exact type and amount of diluent to use.

Essential steps

1. Draw medication into syringe.
2. Further dilute as indicated.
3. Attach filter.

4. Take syringe with medication, patient medication identification card, and anti-infective pledget to bedside.
5. Identify patient.
6. Ascertain patency of infusion.
7. Cleanse flash chamber or side arm of IV tubing with anti-infective pledget.
8. Insert needle, bevel up, at 45-degree angle into center of injection site.

9. Pinch distal tubing 2 to 3 inches above injection site.
10. Inject medication in time recommended.

11. Once administered, remove needle and syringe and unpinch tubing.
12. Regulate IV flow rate.
13. Provide comfort and support to patient.
14. Record all pertinent information (Fig. 4-9).

Key points

Remove all air from syringe, needle, and filter.

Use friction, allow 60-second drying time.
Once entered, realign needle to a 25-degree angle and insert to its hub.

Continually observe patient for expected action and possible reaction.

NURSES' NOTES

Date	Time			Signature
6-1-78	9 AM	Morphine sulfate 5mg in ⊤ ml N.S.	Adm. I.V. Push into in-progress infusion in ⓛ Ant. forearm over	
		R. 18	2 minutes for c/o pain	B. Brown, RN
	9¹⁵/AM	States,	"Pain is relieved."	B. Brown, RN

Fig. 4-9. Nurses' notes recording of intravenous push administration of medication.

DIRECT VENIPUNCTURE METHOD

The purpose of direct venipuncture is to administer an intravenous medication directly into a vein. The volume of fluid may vary from 0.25 to 50 ml.

Essential steps	Key points
1. Select IV site.	
2. Position and tie tourniquet and feel for vein.	
3. Release tourniquet and cleanse site with anti-infective pledget.	Use friction, allow 60-second drying time, avoid contamination of skin after cleansing.
4. Retie tourniquet and feel for vein.	
5. Hold skin taut with thumb below injection site to anchor vein.	
6. Insert needle, bevel up, at 20- to 45-degree angle.	Insert directly over and into vein or along side of vein.
7. Lower hub of needle close to skin for realignment and thrust into vein.	A popping or snapping sound is heard when the vein wall is penetrated; the needle should be on a straight course with the vein; backflow of blood into syringe indicates satisfactory entry.
8. Enter vein slowly.	With slight uplifting motion.
9. Release tourniquet and tension on skin.	
10. Inject medication in time recommended.	Check backflow of blood periodically. Observe patient for expected action and possible reaction
11. Once administered, remove needle and syringe and apply pressure over injection site until bleeding stops.	

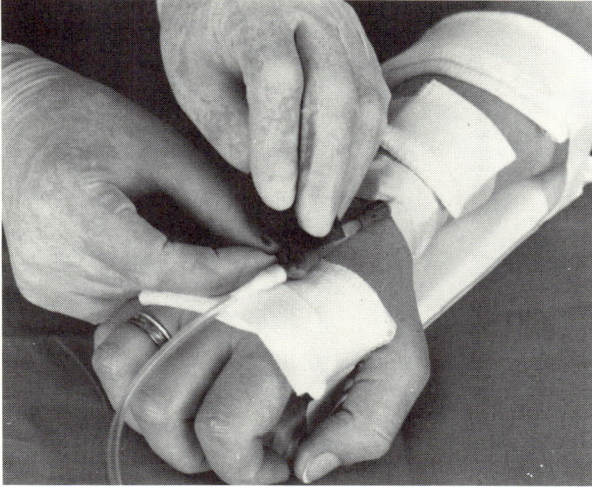

Fig. 4-10. Cleansing of flash chamber prior to intravenous push medication administration into in-progress infusion by way of stainless steel needles and over-the-needle type cannulae during compatible situation. (Courtesy Alton Ochsner Medical Foundation, New Orleans.)

Essential steps	Key points
12. Apply sterile, dry dressing.	A 2 × 2 sponge with 1-inch tape may be used.
13. Provide comfort and support to patient.	
14. Record all pertinent information.	

INTRAVENOUS PUSH INTO IN-PROGRESS INFUSIONS BY WAY OF STAINLESS STEEL NEEDLES AND OVER-THE-NEEDLE TYPE CANNULAE
Compatible situations

Medication to be administered is compatible with in-progress fluid.

Essential steps	Key points
1. Check patency of line.	
2. Cleanse flash chamber or side arm with anti-infective pledget (Fig. 4-10).	Allow 60-second drying time.
3. Pinch tubing and inject medication while timing it.	
4. Unpinch tubing and readjust flow rate.	

Incompatible situations

Medication to be administered is incompatible with in-progress fluid or in-progress fluid is incompatible with medication to be administered.

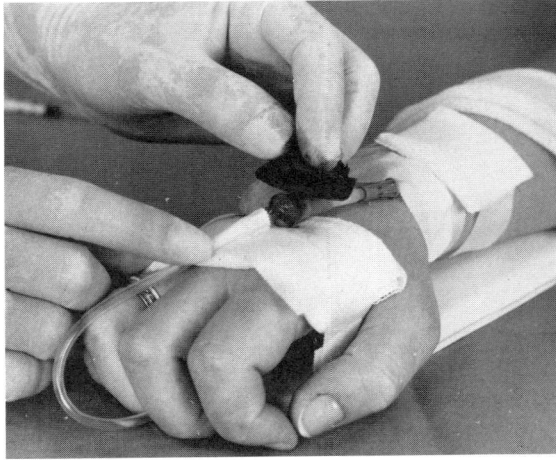

Fig. 4-11. Cleansing of flash chamber prior to intravenous push medication administration into in-progress infusion by way of stainless steel needles and over-the-needle type cannulae during incompatible situation. Larger area of flash chamber is cleansed due to need to insert two needles. (Courtesy Alton Ochsner Medical Foundation, New Orleans.)

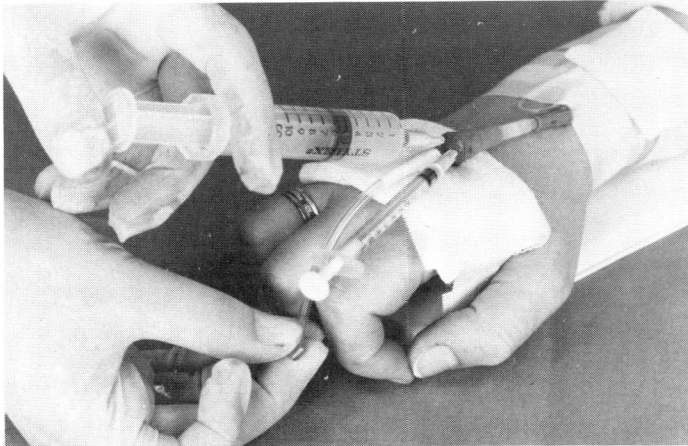

Fig. 4-12. Pushing normal saline to clear tubing of incompatible fluid. (Courtesy Alton Ochsner Medical Foundation, New Orleans.)

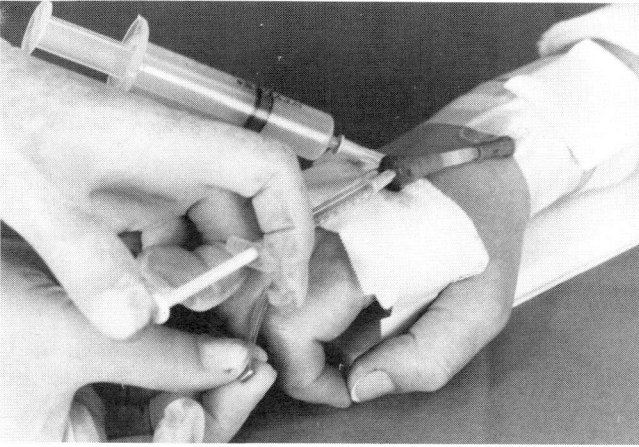

Fig. 4-13. Pushing medication. (Courtesy Alton Ochsner Medical Foundation, New Orleans.)

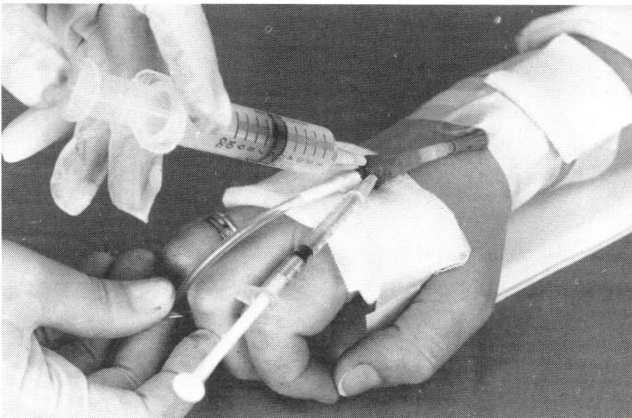

Fig. 4-14. Pushing normal saline to clear tubing of medication prior to resuming in-progress infusion. (Courtesy Alton Ochsner Medical Foundation, New Orleans.)

Essential steps	Key points
1. Check patency of line.	
2. Cleanse flash chamber or side arm with anti-infective pledget (Fig. 4-11).	Allow 60-second drying time. Cleanse larger area, since two needles are to be inserted.
3. Insert needle and syringe containing 5 ml normal saline and needle and syringe containing medication.	
4. Pinch tubing 5 to 7.5 cm (2 to 3 inches) from flash chamber and inject 2.5 ml normal saline (Fig. 4-12).	This clears tubing of incompatible fluid.
5. Inject medication in recommended time (Fig. 4-13).	
6. Inject remaining 2.5 ml normal saline (Fig. 4-14).	Maintain pinch throughout procedure. If flash chamber is used, may inject normal saline in one injection site and medication syringe in another site, avoiding unnecessary removal and reinsertion of normal saline syringe.
7. Unpinch tubing and readjust flow rate.	

INTRAVENOUS PUSH INTO IN-PROGRESS INFUSIONS BY WAY OF IN-THE-NEEDLE TYPE CANNULAE WITH EXTENSION TUBES

IV intrafusors and extension tubes have an average volume of 3.5 ml. This measurement is from injection site to entry into the vein. When medications are pushed through these sets, the length of the tubing must be considered, since the medication must travel the length of the tubing prior to entering the patient's vascular system. This is significant in terms of determining when to begin timing the medication and when to begin making observations regarding the effects of the medication.

Compatible situations

Medication to be administered is compatible with in-progress infusion. (In order to facilitate understanding of this procedure, consider that 1ml of medication is to be administered.)

Essential steps	Key points
1. Check patency of line.	
2. Cleanse flash chamber or side arm with anti-infective pledget.	Allow 60-second drying time.
3. Insert needle and syringe containing 5 ml normal saline and needle and syringe containing medication (1 ml).	
3. Pinch tubing and inject medication.	
4. Inject 2.5 ml normal saline.	Maintain tubing pinch throughout. It is assumed that length of tubing is 3.5 ml. The amount

Essential steps	Key points
	administered thus far assures delivery of the medication to tip of the cannula
5. Inject and time an additional 1 ml of normal saline.	This 1 ml, which is timed, acts as an extension of the medication.
6. Unpinch tubing and readjust flow rate.	

Incompatible situations

Medication to be administered is incompatible with in-progress fluid. (In order to facilitate understanding of this procedure, consider that 1 ml of medication is to be administered.)

Essential steps	Key points
1. Check patency of line.	
2. Cleanse flash chamber or side arm with anti-infective pledget.	Allow 60-second drying time.
3. Insert needle and syringe containing 10 ml normal saline and needle and syringe containing medication (1 ml).	
4. Pinch tubing and inject 5 ml normal saline.	This clears tubing of incompatible fluid.
5. Inject medication.	
6. Inject 2.5 ml normal saline.	Maintain tubing pinch throughout. It is assumed that length of tubing is 3.5 ml. The amount administered thus far assures delivery of the medication to the tip of the cannula.
7. Inject and time an additional 1 ml of normal saline.	This 1 ml, which is timed, acts as an extension of the medication.
8. Use remaining normal saline to flush the tubing and cannula of all medication.	
9. Unpinch tubing and readjust flow rate.	

INTRAVENOUS PUSH INTO INTERMITTENT INFUSION DEVICES—HEPARIN LOCKS
Compatible situations

Medication to be administered is compatible with heparin.

Essential steps	Key points
1. Check patency of line.	
2. Cleanse injection site with anti-infective pledget.	Allow 60-second drying time.
3. Insert syringe and needle containing medication.	Aspirate to ascertain patency.
4. Inject medication in time recommended.	Avoid puncturing soft plastic tubing beyond injection site by using 1-inch or shorter needle.
5. Remove medication syringe and needle.	

Essential steps	Key points
6. Insert syringe and needle containing heparinizing solution.	Heparinizing solution contains 0.1 ml heparin (1000 U/ml) and 0.9 ml normal saline in tuberculin syringe or in unit dose container. This concentration may vary, depending on current practices.
7. Inject 0.5 ml heparinizing solution.	
8. Remove syringe and needle.	

Incompatible situations

Medication to be administered is incompatible with heparin.

Essential steps	Key points
1. Check patency of line.	
2. Cleanse injection site with anti-infective pledget.	Allow 60-second drying time.
3. Insert needle and syringe containing normal saline.	Aspirate to ascertain patency.
4. Inject 0.5 ml normal saline.	This clears tubing of incompatible fluid.
5. Remove normal saline needle and syringe.	
6. Insert needle and syringe containing medication.	
7. Inject medication in time recommended.	Avoid puncturing soft plastic tubing beyond injection site by using 1-inch or shorter needle.
8. Remove medication needle and syringe.	
9. Insert needle and syringe containing normal saline.	
10. Inject 0.5 ml normal saline.	This clears tubing of incompatible medication.
11. Remove normal saline needle and syringe.	
12. Insert syringe and needle containing heparinizing solution.	Heparinizing solution contains 0.1 ml heparin (1000 U/ml) and 0.9 ml normal saline in tuberculin syringe or in unit dose container. This concentration may vary, depending on current practices.
13. Inject 0.5 ml heparinizing solution.	
14. Remove syringe and needle.	

Intravenous piggyback method

The purpose of the intravenous piggyback method is to administer medications intravenously by way of an in-progress infusion. During this intermittent infusion, the medication is diluted in a relatively moderate amount of fluid, usually 10 to 150 ml, an average being 50 to 100 ml, and administered over a 5-minute to 2-hour period.

Methods for piggybacking medications include utilization of burette type tubings, check-valve tubings that function according to the principle of hydrostatic pressure, and straight tubing systems. Each method will be discussed separately.

BURETTE METHOD

Assuming that the infusion has been established, the medication and infusion fluid are compatible, and a burette tubing is attached, the procedure is as follows:

Essential steps	Key points
1. Fill burette with recommended amount of IV fluid	Use fluid from main infusion container.
2. Clamp tubing between main infusion container and burette.	
3. Inject medication into burette by way of its reseal injection site.	
4. Administer medication in time recommended.	Burette airway must be open at this time.
5. Add 10 to 15 ml of fluid to burette from infusion container and administer to patient.	
6. Fill burette with 30 to 40 ml fluid from infusion container.	Close burette airway and open clamp on tubing between main infusion container and burette.
7. The continuous infusion is now reestablished.	

Incompatible situations

Should incompatibility exist between the in-progress infusion and the medication to be administered, a separate infusion container and burette are to be utilized.

This separate system, composed of normal saline or 5% dextrose in water, a burette tubing, and a 22- or 23-gauge needle, is attached to the main or primary infusion set by inserting the needle into the flash chamber or side arm of the primary infusion.

Following flushing the primary tubing with 10 to 15 ml of normal saline or 5% dextrose in water, the medication may be administered using the aforementioned procedure.

The primary system must again be flushed following administration of the medication. The primary system is shut off during the medication administration.

CHECK-VALVE TUBING SYSTEM METHOD

A check-valve tubing system is composed of a primary and secondary tubing (Fig. 4-15).

The primary tubing is connected to the primary fluid container, which is usually an in-progress infusion. Its tubing contains a check

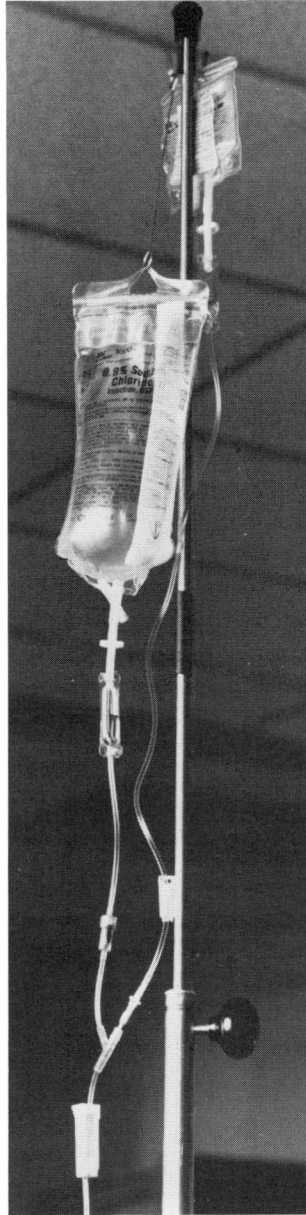

Fig. 4-15. Check valve tubing system with primary and secondary fluid containers and tubings. (Courtesy Alton Ochsner Medical Foundation, New Orleans.)

valve that moves up or down to open or close the tube. Hydrostatic pressure determines movement of the check valve.

The secondary tubing is connected to the secondary fluid container, which contains the medication to be administered.

Essential steps	Key points
1. Add medication to secondary infusion container.	Volume of container is 50 to 100 ml.
2. Label with date, time, patient's name, room number, medication added, dosage, and admixer's name.	
3. Attach secondary tubing with needle and prime.	
4. Lower primary infusion container 6 to 8 inches below secondary container.	
5. Attach secondary container to primary container.	By inserting secondary container needle to side arm of primary container tubing.
6. Open secondary tubing clamp.	
7. Regulate rate of flow with primary tubing clamp.	
8. After medication administration, clamp secondary tubing and raise primary infusion container.	
9. Regulate flow rate.	
10. Record all pertinent information.	

Incompatible situations

Should incompatibility exist between the in-progress infusion and the medication to be administered, a separate system is used. The procedure is much like that of the burette method in that a separate system is piggybacked to the in-progress infusion, the in-progress infusion is shut off, flushed, medication administered, flushed, and then the in-progress infusion reestablished.

STRAIGHT TUBING SYSTEM METHOD

The straight tubing method uses a straight tubing that is attached to the medication container. The medication is attached to the in-progress infusion by piggyback.

The in-progress infusion is referred to as the primary system and the medication container as the secondary system.

Essential steps	Key points
1. Add medication to secondary container and label as previously described.	
2. Attach tubing and needle and prime.	
3. Insert needle into flash chamber or side arm of the primary system tubing.	
4. Clamp primary infusion.	

NURSES' NOTES

Date	Time			Signature
6-1-78	9 AM	Ancef 500 mg in	Adm. I.V.P.B. into	
		50 ml D5.9 saline sol	in-progress infusion	
			in (L) Ant. forearm	
			over 30 minutes.	B. Brown, RN
	9 45/AM		Sitting in chair et	
			Conversing c̄ wife	B. Brown, RN

Fig. 4-16. Nurses' notes recording of intravenous piggyback administration of medication.

Essential steps

5. Open secondary infusion.
6. Administer medication in time recommended.
7. Reestablish and regulate flow of primary infusion.
8. Remove secondary system.
9. Record all pertinent information (Fig. 4-16).

Key points

Incompatible situations

Should incompatibilities exist, it is recommended that the primary tubing be flushed with normal saline or another appropriate fluid before the medication is delivered and before the in-progress infusion is reestablished.

References

Del Bueno, D. J., et al.: Teaching pharmacology, Nurs. Outlook, **19**:6, 1971.

Francke, D.: Handbook of I.V. additive review, Drug intelligence publication, Hamilton, Ill., 1973, The Hamilton Press.

Gahart, B.: Intravenous medications—a handbook for nurses and other allied health personnel, ed. 2, St. Louis, 1977, The C. V. Mosby Co.

Plumer, A.: Principles and practice of intravenous therapy, ed. 2, Boston, 1975, Little, Brown & Co.

Rodman, M., and Smith, D.: Clinical pharmacology in nursing, Philadelphia, 1974, J. B. Lippincott Co.

Thomas, C., editor: Taber's cyclopedic medical dictionary, ed. 13, Philadelphia, 1977, F. A. Davis Co.

Chapter 5

Intravenous fluids

Prior to the 1920s, sheep's blood, cod liver oil, and milk were administered intravenously. These primitive attempts at supplying fluid, nutrition, electrolytes, and vitamins were soon abandoned, since side effects proved serious and often fatal.

Sterile intravenous fluids that resembled fluids used today were initially prepared by individual hospitals. During the 1930s fluids were (and continue to be) manufactured by commercial companies. Standards for fluid content, pH, containers, preparation techniques, sterility, and stability were established by the United States Food and Drug Administration. These standards continue to be adhered to.

With the discovery of antibiotics during World War II, the value of multiple component therapy, fluids and electrolytes, or polytherapy was realized (Kabat, 1971). Problems related to incompatibilities of multiple component therapy caused a reverting to plain fluids in the 1970s.

Until the 1950s, administration of intravenous therapy was the responsibility of the physician or a technician trained and supervised by the physician.

At the start, intravenous fluids were administered by syringe and needle. Because of the dangers of infection and air embolism inherent in this technique, the utilization of glass reservoirs replaced this first method.

Advances in dialysis, intensive care, coronary care, and oncologic nursing, and the general increase in the use of the vascular system as a route of administering intravenous fluids and medications charges the nurse with the responsibility of having in-depth knowledge and understanding of the vascular system and its compartments, fluid and electrolyte balance, and acid-base balance.

No longer can the nurse merely hang a fluid, regulate it, and record that the therapy was administered as ordered by the physician. The nurse must also be able to recognize signs and symptoms of fluid and electrolyte normals, deficits, and overloads. The chemical nature of solutions, incompatibilities, and osmolarity (hypotonicity, isotonicity, and hypertonicity) must be understood. Fluid and electrolyte balance, acid-base balance and its effects, blood levels of electrolytes, and changes in ECG patterns are all important considerations.

FLUID AND ELECTROLYTE BALANCE

Body cells and tissues are nurtured as arterioles and venules exchange nutrients, oxygen, and carbon dioxide at the cellular level. For exchange to occur, pressures within the capillary walls and cellular membranes must be at a certain point. Pressures are determined by the presence of certain electrolytes, especially sodium and potassium, and certain gases, especially oxygen and carbon dioxide. A similar situation exists between oxygen and carbon dioxide within the alveolar sacs in the lungs.

Substances are transported through the cell membrane by diffusion, osmosis, and active transport.

Diffusion is the process whereby there is a tendency for molecules of a substance, because of their incessant motion, to move from a region of higher concentration to one of lower concentration, even if aqueous solutions of different materials stand in contact. Mixing occurs on standing even if the solutions are separated by thin membranes.

Osmosis, a related process, is the passage of a solvent through a selectively permeable membrane, separating solutions of different concentrations. The solvent, usually water, passes through the membrane from the region of lower concentration of solute to that of higher concentration of solute, thus tending to equalize the concentration of the two solutions. The rate of osmosis depends on the difference in osmotic pressure of the solutions on the two sides of the membrane, the permeability of the membrane, the electrical potential across the membrane, and the electrical charge on the walls of the membrane pores.

Osmotic pressure develops because of the differing concentrations of solutions on either side of the membrane. Osmotic pressure varies with varying concentrations of the two solutions and with temperature increases (Thomas, 1977).

Active transport is the movement of materials across the cell membranes by means of a carrier. The difference between active transport and diffusion is that active transport requires energy so that transport can occur against a concentration gradient or against an electrical or pressure gradient (Guyton, 1976).

The vascular system is divided into two main compartments: the intracellular (within the cells) and extracellular (outside the cells). The extracellular compartment is further divided into the plasma, blood vessles, and interstitial compartments or divisions.

A third compartment can be considered: the transcellular compartment. This includes fluid and electrolytes found outside the other two compartments and may be classified as the fluid and electrolytes from certain secreting and excreting organs and tissues such as the gastro-intestinal secretions, urine, and products of cellular metabolism. The function and composition of the transcellular fluid differs from the extracellular fluid. Most often the fluid in this compartment is considered to be part of the extracellular compartment.

There are approximately 75 trillion cells within the intracellular compartment of a normal average adult (68 kg or 150 lb). Of the 40 liters of fluid within the body, 25 liters are inside the intracellular compartment.

The total amount of fluid within the extracellular compartment is approximately 15 liters. The extracellular fluid is divided into interstitial fluid (fluid around the cells), the plasma, which exchanges freely with the interstitial fluid by way of diffusion through the pores of the capillaries, the cerebrospinal fluid, the intraocular fluid, and the fluid in potential spaces such as the visceral and parietal spaces, peritoneal cavity, pericardial cavity, joint spaces, and bursae (Guyton, 1976).

The total amount of water in the normal average adult ranges from 45% to 70% of total body fluid. The precise percentage depends on the amount of adipose tissue present, since fat is relatively free of water. The fluid distribution is usually two-thirds in the intracellular compartment and one-third in the extracellular compartment (McGaw, 1963).

The average blood volume of a normal adult is 5000 ml, with 3000 ml being plasma and 2000 ml being red blood cells. This average volume varies among individuals. Age, sex, and weight are factors that determine the variations (Guyton, 1976).

A fluid is a nonsolid liquid or gaseous substance (Thomas, 1977).

A solution is a liquid containing dissolved substances. The liquid portion of a solution is called the solvent, while the substance dissolved in the liquid is called the solute. The strength of the substance dissolved is determined by the amount of solute present within the solvent and is represented by ratio, percentage, or grains to the ounce.

Normal body fluids are composed of nonelectrolytes and electrolyte solutes. Nonelectrolyte solutes remain intact and therefore do not ionize in water. Examples are glucose, urea, and creatinine. Electrolyte solutes do ionize in water and therefore break into electrically charged particles called ions. Ions are classified as cations, or those that are posi-

Table 1. Composition of intracellular and extracellular fluid

Substance	Extracellular	Intracellular
Sodium (Na$^+$)	142 mEq/liter	10 mEq/liter
Potassium (K$^+$)	5 mEq/liter	141 mEq/liter
Calcium (Ca^{++})	5 mEq/liter	1 mEq/liter
Magnesium (Mg^{++})	3 mEq/liter	58 mEq/liter
Chloride (Cl$^-$)	103 mEq/liter	4 mEq/liter
Bicarbonate (HCo$_3^-$)	28 mEq/liter	10 mEq/liter
Phosphates	4 mEq/liter	75 mEq/liter
Sulfate (So$_4^{--}$)	1 mEq/liter	2 mEq/liter
Glucose	90 mg/100 ml	0-20 mg/100 ml
Amino acids	30 mg/100 ml	200 mg/100 ml
Cholesterol	—	—
Phospholipids	0.5 g/100 ml	2-95 g/100 ml
Neutral fat	—	—

tively charged, and anions, or those that are negatively charged. Examples of cations are sodium, potassium, calcium, and magnesium. Examples of anions are bicarbonate and chloride.

Under normal conditions electrolyte solutes are balanced so that there is equal distribution of cations and anions. The concentration of particles is expressed as milliequivalents per milliliter (mEq/ml).

Fluid in each compartment has a distinct electrolyte pattern within the intracellular and extracellular compartment, as seen in Table 1. This pattern is maintained by the processes of cellular metabolism. Since water moves freely from one compartment to the other, an osmotic equilibrium is maintained. Should the extracellular electrolyte concentration increase, water diffuses from the intracellular compartment to the extracellular compartment, thereby increasing cellular tonicity and diluting the extracellular compartment and vice versa.

Osmolality of a solution is determined by the concentration of ions in that solution. This concentration determines osmotic pressure. To express the concentration of ions in a solution in terms of osmolality, the unit, called osmol, is used in place of grams. One osmol is the number of particles in one gram molecular weight of undissociated solute and is the unit for osmotic pressure. One thousandth of an osmol is the milliosmol.

The presence of water causes electrolytes to become electrically charged. This occurs when the molecules of the electrolytes split into ions.

Table 2. Cation and anion concentration in the intracellular, interstitial, and plasma fluid*

Cations			Anions		
Intracellular					
Na$^+$	15 mEq		HCO$_3^-$	10 mEq	
K$^+$	150 mEq		Cl$^-$	1 mEq	
Ca^{++}	2 mEq		HPO$_4^{--}$	100 mEq	
Mg^{++}	27 mEq		SO$_4^{--}$	20 mEq	
			Protein	63 mEq	
TOTAL	194 mEq			194 mEq	
Interstitial					
Na$^+$	147 mEq		HCO$_3^-$	30 mEq	
K$^+$	4 mEq		Cl$^-$	114 mEq	
Ca^{++}	2.5 mEq		HPO$_4^{--}$	2 mEq	
Mg^{++}	1 mEq		SO$_4^{--}$	1 mEq	
			Org. Ac.	7.5 mEq	
			Protein	0 mEq	
TOTAL	154.5 mEq			154.5 mEq	
Plasma					
Na$^+$	142 mEq		HCO$_3^-$	24 mEq	
K$^+$	5 mEq		Cl$^-$	105 mEq	
Ca^{++}	5 mEq		HPO$_4^{--}$	2 mEq	
Mg^{++}	2 mEq		SO$_4^{--}$	1 mEq	
			Org. Ac.	6 mEq	
			Protein	16 mEq	
TOTAL	154 mEq			154 mEq	

*Note that each fluid compartment is different in terms of the electrolyte composition and concentration. In addition, the volume of water is different. The main difference between the interstitial and plasma fluid is the presence of protein in the plasma. Changes in water volume can alter electrolyte patterns and changes in electrolytes can change the water volume. Electrolytes can be related to water distribution, osmotic pressure, neuromuscular irritability, and acid-base balance.

Cations tend to unite with anions, producing solutes (also termed salts or minerals) such as sodium chloride, calcium sulfate, and the like (Baxter, 1972).

In order that balance be maintained there must be an equal number of cations and anions present within the body at all times.

The unit of measure for electrolytes is the milliequivalent (mEq). One mEq of any cation is able to react with one mEq of any anion.

Table 2 shows the cation and anion concentration in the intracellular, interstitial, and plasma fluid.

PURPOSE OF ELECTROLYTES
Cations
SODIUM

Sodium is the major electrolyte in the extracellular fluid. It controls water distribution within the intracellular and extracellular compartments. Water has an affinity for sodium and, as such, wherever sodium is, water goes. When the body levels of sodium are elevated, water levels are elevated and vice versa. This tends to cause either edema or dehydration.

Elevated concentrations of sodium within the plasma stimulate the secretion of antidiuretic hormone (ADH), thereby allowing water to be retained by the renal tubules. This allows for adequate dilution of sodium. Low concentrations of sodium within the plasma retards or prevents secretion of ADH, thereby allowing water to be excreted by the renal tubules. Retardation of renal function leads to a rise in blood urea nitrogen, which delays excretion of water and salts.

The plasma bicarbonate varies directly with intracellular sodium in that sodium enters the cells when there has been a loss of intracellular potassium.

POTASSIUM

Potassium is the major electrolyte of the intracellular fluid. Potassium can be lifesaving or detrimental. It is necessary for cellular activity. When cells die, potassium enters the extracellular fluid and sodium enters the cell. This also occurs during altered metabolic activity within the cells. The entrance of potassium into the cells is dependent on normal metabolism and glucose utilization. The kidneys do not conserve potassium. Increased levels of potassium result in loss of sodium and decreased levels of potassium result in retention of sodium.

CALCIUM

Calcium provides the framework for bones and teeth. When ionized, calcium plays a role in the normal blood-clotting mechanism and regulation of neuromuscular irritability. It has a sedative effect on the cells of the nervous system. Without adequate amounts of protein, calcium is not utilized. Vitamin D assists with the utilization of calcium.

Calcium is not completely absorbed from the gastrointestinal tract. The digestive juices secrete 5 to 10 mg of calcium per 100 ml. A negative calcium balance occurs when absorption is inhibited within the gastrointestinal tract and when calcium intake is low.

Parathyroid hormones control the calcium-phosphorus ratio. Ionization of calcium is depressed in states of metabolic alkalosis.

MAGNESIUM

Magnesium plays a role in the metabolism of carbohydrates and protein by exerting enzyme activity. Approximately 35% of the available magnesium is bound to protein. Magnesium, like calcium, is involved in the regulation of neuromuscular irritability.

Magnesium is present in bones and teeth. The absorption of magnesium is similar to that of calcium.

Magnesium and potassium influence the deposition of protein (Baxter, 1972). There is an acceleration of magnesium exchange within the tissues when dextrose and insulin are administered parenterally. Experimental studies indicate that magnesium may have an influence on controlling certain cardiac arrhythmias, including those caused by digitalis intoxication.

Anions
BICARBONATE

The concentration of bicarbonate is related to renal function. The kidneys regulate the amount of cations available to combine with bicarbonate. Women have approximately 2.5 mEq/liter less bicarbonate than men. Bicarbonate is present as a result of metabolism and the production of carbon dioxide.

CHLORIDE

Chloride acts as a buffer during the exchange of carbon dioxide for oxygen within the red blood cells. During the oxygenation process, chloride shifts out of the red blood cells into the plasma and bicarbonate enters the red blood cells from the plasma. This results in venous blood having lower concentrations of chloride than arterial blood. In addition, during the process of oxygenation, the red blood cells become relatively dehydrated.

Women have approximately 2.5 mEq/liter more chloride than do men. The greatest percentage of chloride is found in the interstitial fluid and lymphatic fluid. A deficiency in chloride results in a deficiency in potassium, and an excess of chloride results in an excess of potassium. Chloride losses usually follow sodium losses. This mechanism varies, since a chloride loss is compensated for by an increase in bicarbonate, which leads to preservation of osmotic pressure and water balance. Changes in acid-base balance reflect changes in chloride concentrations (Baxter, 1972).

PHOSPHATE

Phosphate is the major anion within the cells, and it may be expressed as phosphorus (Baxter, 1972). Approximately 95% of all phosphorus is reabsorbed by the renal tubules. The rate of reabsorption by the renal tubules is increased by vitamin D. This is not so regarding phosphorus reabsorption by the gastrointestinal tract.

The metabolism of phosphorus is directly related to calcium. The amount of phosphorus and calcium present is related to dietary intake, acid-base regulation, and endocrine regulation (Baxter, 1972).

SULFATE

Sulfate is related to cellular protein. Excretion of this electrolyte is retarded during periods of renal insufficiency.

ORGANIC SALTS

The organic salts (lactic acid, pyruvate, acetoacetate, and citrate) play a role in cellular metabolism. The main organic salt is lactic acid. Lactic acid displaces bicarbonate. Lactic acid levels rise during hyperventilation and when patients are receiving infusions of glucose and bicarbonate.

PROTEINATE

Proteinate assists the osmotic mechanism when substances move from the interstitial fluid into the capillaries.

	Intake				Output		
Time	PO	TF	IV	Blood	Urine	Suction	Other
7-3	600 ml	0	D5W 1000 ml	WB 500 ml	1900 ml	0	0
3-11	700 ml	0	D5 RL 1000 ml	R.B.C. 250 ml	1400 ml	N.G. 200 ml	0
			D5W 100 ml				
11-7	200 ml	0	D5 RL 1000 ml	0	1000 ml	150 ml	0
			D5W 100 ml				
Total	1500 ml	0	3200 ml	750 ml	4300 ml	350 ml	0
24 hr Total	4700 ml			700 ml	4650 ml		

Fig. 5-1. Intake and output record (8 and 24 hours). Transfusion intake is included here; however, 8- and 24-hour totals of transfusions are kept separate from all other intake totals.

ABNORMALITIES OF FLUID AND ELECTROLYTE BALANCE

Recognition of losses or overloads of fluids and electrolytes is accomplished through assessment of objective and subjective symptoms and analysis of laboratory data.

Accurate records of intake and output and daily weights of the patient serve as valuable guides in determining balance or imbalance (Figs. 5-1 and 5-2).

Sources of fluid and electrolyte output are lacrimation, vomitus, respiration, perspiration, bronchorrhea, salivation, lactation, burn and wound exudate, gastric and chest suction, diarrhea, urine, and draining fistulae.

Output is categorized as sensible and insensible. Clearly stated, sensible losses are losses that can be measured, while insensible losses are those that cannot be measured.

Examples of deficits and overloads related to fluids and electrolytes follow.

Time	PO	TF	IV	Blood	Urine	Suction	Other
7A	O	O	100 ml	100 ml	30 ml	O	O
8	O	O	100 ml	100 ml	50 ml	30 ml	O
9	O	O	100 ml	50 ml	80 ml	10 ml	O
10	O	O	100 ml	O	90 ml	10 ml	O
11	O	O	100 ml	O	90 ml	O	O
12N	O	O	100 ml	O	90 ml	O	O
1	O	O	100 ml	O	60 ml	10 ml	O
2	O	O	100 ml	O	60 ml	O	O
Total	—O—	—O—	—800 ml—	—250 ml—	—550 ml—	—60 ml—	—O—
3P	O	O	100 ml	O	150 ml	20 ml	O
4	O	O	125 ml	O	150 ml	10 ml	O
5	O	O	125 ml	O	100 ml	40 ml	O
6	O	O	125 ml	O	100 ml	10 ml	O
7	O	O	125 ml	O	100 ml	10 ml	O
8	O	O	125 ml	O	100 ml	O	O
9	O	O	125 ml	O	100 ml	O	O
10	O	O	125 ml	O	100 ml	20 ml	O
Total	—O—	—O—	—975 ml—	—O—	—900 ml—	—110 ml—	—O—
11	O	O	125 ml	100 ml	150 ml	10 ml	O
12MN	O	O	125 ml	100 ml	150 ml	O	O
1	O	O	125 ml	100 ml	100 ml	O	O
2	O	O	125 ml	100 ml	100 ml	O	O
3	O	O	125 ml	100 ml	100 ml	O	O
4	O	O	125 ml	O	100 ml	O	O
5	O	O	125 ml	O	100 ml	10 ml	O
6A	O	O	125 ml	O	100 ml	O	O
Total	—O—	—O—	—1000 ml—	—500 ml—	—900 ml—	—20 ml—	—O—
Grand total	O	O	2775 ml	750 ml	2350 ml	190 ml	O

Fig. 5-2. Hourly intake and output record.

Volume deficit

Volume deficit occurs when there is an inadequate intake during such states as nausea, vomiting, diarrhea, excessive drainage from fistulae and wounds, intestinal obstruction, severe burns, lymphatic edema, and ascites. A volume deficit may also be produced by diabetes insipidus.

Signs and symptoms include thirst, weight loss, hypotension, oliguria, lassitude, poor skin turgor, dry skin and mucous membranes, furrows on the tongue, lowered body temperature, and tachycardia.

Laboratory findings include an elevated erythrocyte count, elevated hematocrit and hemoglobin, elevated urine specific gravity, azotemia, and in cases of sodium depletion, the urine may lack sodium and chloride (Brunner and Suddarth, 1975; McGaw, 1963).

Volume excess (overhydration)

Volume excess, or overhydration, includes conditions where excessive quantities of isotonic solutions such as normal saline have been administered, follows excessive sodium chloride or electrolyte intake, and occurs with congestive heart failure and renal and hepatic diseases. A hypotonic volume excess may be caused by fluid overloading in excess of sodium.

Signs and symptoms include shortness of breath, generalized edema with weight gain, and pulmonary congestion.

Laboratory findings include decreased erythrocyte, hematocrit, and hemoglobin counts, hyponatremia, hypochloremia, oliguria, and lowered urine specific gravity. Specific gravity of urine in volume deficit would be elevated, indicating concentrated urine, since volume excess many times is caused by renal disease or congestive heart failure and other conditions that cause a decreased production of urine.

Total electrolyte concentration deficit

Total electrolyte concentration deficit occurs when the water intake exceeds output such as that which occurs during states of adrenal insufficiency; malnutrition; cardiac, renal, and hepatic disease; and when water is replaced without adequate electrolyte replacement. States of hyponatremia, potassium depletion, and excessive secretion of ADH are present.

Signs and symptoms include headache, apprehension, nausea, abdominal cramping, hyperactive reflexes, confusion, polyuria, oliguria, and hypotension.

Laboratory findings reveal a plasma sodium level below 130 mEq/liter and concentrated urine due to water retention.

Total electrolyte concentration excess

Total electrolyte concentration excess occurs following inadequate water intake, especially during fever, diarrhea, excessive sweating, and diabetes insipidus.

Signs and symptoms include thirst, oliguria, weakness, excitement, dry mucous membranes, tachycardia, and fever.

Laboratory findings reveal a plasma sodium level exceeding 147 mEq/liter and urine specific gravity greater than 1.026 (McGaw, 1963).

Sodium deficit (hyponatremia, low-sodium syndrome, electrolyte concentration deficit, or hypotonic dehydration)

Sodium deficit occurs during states of decreased intake or increased output of sodium or during states of increased intake or decreased output of water. Causative factors include heat exhaustion, renal disease where sodium is lost rather than retained, gastric suctioning, tap water enemas, potent diuretic therapy, parenteral administration of electrolyte-free solutions, and fresh-water drowning.

Signs and symptoms include apprehension, abdominal cramping, convulsions, oliguria or anuria, hypotension, rapid thready pulse, cold clammy skin, and cyanosis.

Laboratory findings reveal a plasma sodium level less than 137 mEq/liter, chloride level less than 98 mEq/liter, and urine specific gravity less than 1.010 (Brunner and Suddarth, 1975; McGaw, 1963).

Sodium excess (hypernatremia, hypertonic dehydration, salt excess, or oversalting)

The causative factors of sodium excess include a decreased water intake and an increased sodium intake, rapid breathing with excessive water loss through the lungs, profuse water diarrhea, and salt-water drowning.

Signs and symptoms include dry, sticky mucous membranes, flushed skin, thirst, oliguria and anuria, and elevated temperature.

Laboratory findings reveal a plasma sodium level in excess of 147 mEq/liter, chloride level greater than 106 mEq/liter, and a urine specific gravity in excess of 1.030 (McGaw, 1963).

Potassium deficit (hypokalemia)

Both intracellular and extracellular potassium deficits are caused by potassium loss without replacement. Causative factors include vomiting, diarrhea, gastric suction, draining fistulae, prolonged diuretic and steroid therapy, diabetic acidosis, and the use of dextrose solutions with insulin, which may cause rapid deposition of glycogen.

Signs and symptoms include muscle cramps, lethargy, irritability, distension, and cardiac arrhythmias.

The effects of potassium deficit on the heart include depression of the ST segment, prolongation of the QT interval, and a low, broad T wave. Severe depletion produces premature ventricular contractions, partial AV block, and auricular fibrillations, especially in patients receiving digitalis.

Laboratory findings reveal a potassium level less than 3 to 4 mEq/liter. The potassium plasma level may be normal during periods where the intracellular level is deficient (Brunner and Suddarth, 1975; McGaw, 1963).

Potassium excess (hyperkalemia)

Potassium excess occurs in renal disease, adrenal insufficiency, excessive administration of potassium, and with excessive shifts of potassium following burns and crushing injuries.

Signs and symptoms include paresthesia, listlessness, confusion, weakness, heaviness of legs, and flaccid paralysis. The electrocardiogram shows elevated T waves, depressed ST segment, decreased size of the R wave, and increased S component with disappearance of P waves and spread of QRS and T waves.

Laboratory findings reveal a plasma potassium level greater than 6 mEq/liter (Brunner and Suddarth, 1975; McGaw, 1963).

Calcium deficit (hypocalcemia)

Calcium deficit occurs because of conditions such as sprue, steatorrhea, acute pancreatitis, massive subcutaneous infection, generalized peritonitis, hypoparathyroidism, chronic renal disease, excessive administration of citrated blood, inadequate intake of calcium, and vitamin D deficiency.

Signs and symptoms include tingling of the fingers, tetany, muscle cramps, carpopedal spasms, convulsions, laryngeal stridor, and prolonged QT interval.

Laboratory findings reveal a calcium level greater than 4.5 mEq/liter. An electrocardiogram, x-ray films, and total protein concentration determinations are necessary diagnostic studies.

Calcium excess (hypercalcemia)

Calcium excess occurs in conditions such as hyperparathyroidism, multiple myeloma, multiple fractures, prolonged immoblization, excessive intake of vitamin D and calcium, sarcoidosis, and skeletal malignancies.

Signs and symptoms include nausea, vomiting, lost muscle tone, flank pain if renal calculi are present, bone pain, and osteoporosis with resultant pathologic fractures.

Laboratory findings reveal a calcium level greater than 5.8 mEq/liter. The electrocardiogram and x-ray films are necessary diagnostic studies (Brunner and Suddarth, 1975; McGaw, 1963).

Protein deficit (hypoproteinemia or protein malnutrition)

Protein deficit occurs following blood loss, deficient intake of protein in the diet, draining wounds, severe trauma, fractures, and burns.

Signs and symptoms include fatigue, pallor, decreased muscle mass and tone, depression, weight loss, and decreased resistance to infection.

Laboratory findings reveal a plasma albumin level less than 4.0 g/100 ml. Erythrocyte, hematocrit, and hemoglobin counts are decreased (Brunner and Suddarth, 1975; McGaw, 1963).

Magnesium deficit (hypomagnesemia)

Magnesium deficit is a condition that can be mistaken for potassium deficit. It occurs in alcoholism, cirrhosis of the liver, malnutrition, anorexia, vomiting, diarrhea, and prolonged intravenous administration of magnesium-free solutions when there is no other source for this element to enter the body (Brunner and Suddarth, 1975; McGaw, 1963).

Magnesium excess (hypermagnesemia)

Magnesium excess occurs following repeated enemas with magnesium sulfate (epsom salts) and magnesium sulfate overdose in chronic constipation.

Signs and symptoms include a curare-like paralysis, hypotension, sedation, and asystole.

Laboratory findings reveal an elevated magnesium plasma level (Brunner and Suddarth, 1975; McGaw, 1963).

ACID-BASE BALANCE

Taber's Cyclopedic Medical Dictionary (1977) defines acid-base balance as the "mechanism by which the acids and alkalis are kept in a state of equilibrium so that the hydrogen ion concentration of the arterial blood is maintained at an approximate pH of 7.35 to 7.45."

The pH of venous blood is 7.35 because of the carbon dioxide present that forms carbonic acid in this fluid. The pH of the intracellular fluid is 7. It ranges from 4.5 to 7.4.

Acid-base balance is accomplished by the action of buffering systems of the blood and homeostatic functions of the cardiovascular, respiratory, urinary, and endocrine systems. Disturbances in acid-base balance result in either acidosis or alkalosis.

The degree of acidity or alkalinity of a substance is expressed in pH values.

The pH scale is as follows:

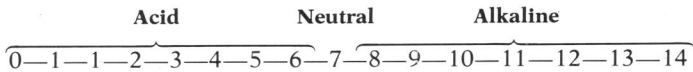

Acid	Neutral	Alkaline

0—1—1—2—3—4—5—6—7—8—9—10—11—12—13—14

The number 7 on the scale represents a neutral state. All numbers less than 7 are considered to be within the acid range, while all numbers greater than 7 are considered to be within the alkaline range. Each number on the scale represents a logarithm, hence there is a ten-fold difference between each unit. For example, pH 5 is 10 times as acid as pH 6, and pH 4 is 100 times as acid as pH 6 (Thomas, 1977; Plumer, 1975).

Buffering systems

There are three main body fluid buffer systems. The carbonate-bicarbonate buffer, the phosphate buffer, and the protein buffer. These chemical systems function to maintain pH by maintaining the hydrogen ion concentration (Guyton, 1976).

The *carbonate-bicarbonate buffer system* works in the following manner: carbonate ions react with hydrogen to produce bicarbonate ions, or the bicarbonate ion may react with hydrogen to form carbonic acid. Removal of excess hydrogen ions tends to keep the pH constant. If hydroxyl ions are introduced, they will be neutralized by hydrogen ions produced by the dissociation of carbonic acid. Thus the carbonate-bicarbonate buffer system can neutralize excess hydrogen or hydroxyl ions. This system buffers effectively around pH 7.0 (Johnson, 1972).

The *phosphate system* buffers effectively around pH 7.2. Phosphate is a salt of phosphoric acid. Monosodium phosphate, an acid, and disodium phosphate, an alkali, are present in low concentrations in the blood. This system functions in a fashion similar to the carbonate-bicarbonate system, but it is composed of salts of phosphoric acid.

The *protein buffer system* is the most powerful buffering system in the body. Three-fourths of all the chemical buffering power of body fluids is intracellular, and most of this buffering results from intracellular proteins. The protein buffering system works in exactly the same manner as does the carbonate-bicarbonate system (Guyton, 1976).

Homeostatic regulation

The cardiovascular, respiratory, urinary, and endocrine (adrenal, pituitary, and parathyroid glands) systems serve to regulate homeostasis of fluid and electrolytes, osmolality, and acid-base balance.

The cardiovascular and urinary systems regulate the amount and composition of urine. Imbalances occur during failure of these systems and during disease processes, shock, postoperative stress, and alarm reactions (McGaw, 1963).

The mineralocorticoid hormone, aldosterone, secreted by the adrenal cortex, regulates the metabolism of sodium, chloride, and potassium. Aldosterone increases the resorption of sodium bicarbonate from the renal tubules. During stress, an increased secretion of aldosterone occurs, further increasing the resorption of sodium bicarbonate. During conditions of adrenal insufficiency there is a loss of sodium, and during conditions of adrenal hyperactivity there is excessive retention of sodium.

The antidiuretic hormone (ADH) is secreted by the posterior lobe of the pituitary gland. ADH increases water resorption in the distal tubule of the kidney. During states of increased body fluid osmolality, decreased fluid volume, shock, and stress an increased amount of ADH is secreted. During states of decreased osmolality, increased fluid volume, and with the presence of alcohol the secretion of ADH decreases. The result is an increased excretion of dilute urine (McGaw, 1963).

The extracellular concentration of calcium and phosphate is regulated by the parathyroid glands. Hyperparathyroidism causes an elevated calcium level and a depressed phosphate level (McGaw, 1963).

Pulmonary ventilatory capacity to remove carbon dioxide determines regulation of acid-base balance, since the conversion of carbonic acid to carbon dioxide and water eliminates hydrogen ions. During states of hyperventilation excessive carbon dioxide is exhaled, thereby depleting hydrogen ions and causing respiratory alkalosis. During hypoventilation carbon dioxide, carbonic acid, and hydrogen ions are in excess, producing respiratory acidosis.

Under normal circumstances the kidney retains or eliminates in order to maintain a state of equilibrium. This selective capacity of the kidney is impaired during certain disease processes; stress; debilitating disorders; and cardiovascular, renal, adrenal, and hepatic conditions.

During certain disease states, excessive sodium and water may be retained, causing a hypotonic overexpansion of body fluid that is generally difficult to correct—far more difficult, in fact, than the opposing condition of dehydration.

The administration of fluids and electrolytes serves to correct and maintain balance. This can be accomplished over a period of several days of intravenous fluid and electrolyte therapy. Once the imbalance is at least partially corrected, the body's own compensatory mechanism may complement the therapy.

OSMOLALITY

Osmolality represents the total water and solute concentration of a solution (Plumer, 1975).

A solution with one osmol of solute dissolved in each kilogram of water is said to have 1 osmol/kg, and a solution with 1/1000 of an osmol per kilogram is said to have 1 milliosmol (mOsm)/kg (Guyton, 1976).

The normal osmolality of the extracellular and intracellular fluid is approximately 300 mOsm/kg.

Osmolarity expresses the number of osmols per liter of solution rather than osmols per kilogram.

Although osmolality determines the rate of osmosis, the difference in quantity of osmolality and osmolarity is less than 1%. The term osmolarity may be more commonly used because of its practicality in terms of liters versus kilograms.

Isotonic solutions such as plasma and normal saline contain approximately 290 mOsm/liter. A solution is considered hypotonic when the milliosmol concentration is less than 240 mOsm/liter of an isotonic solution of plasma. A solution is considered hypertonic when the milliosmol concentration is greater than 340 mOsm/liter of an isotonic solution of plasma (Plumer, 1975). The total milliosmol concentration per liter is the sum of milliosmols per liter of each ionized and nonionized compound in a given solution.

Since there is a direct relationship between the concentration of electrolytes in intracellular and extracellular fluid, analysis of plasma electrolyte levels and patient symptoms serves as a guide in determining disturbances. However, because of rates of shifts of electrolytes between the two compartments, plasma analysis may be misleading, since the plasma levels may show highs or lows while the intracellular values may be different.

Electrolytes serve to control water volume through osmotic pressure and to maintain acid-base balance (Plumer, 1975).

ABNORMALITIES OF ACID-BASE BALANCE

Acid-base disturbances may be produced by deficits or excesses of bicarbonate or carbonic acid due to alterations in the hydrogen ion concentration in the extracellular fluid.

In order for the hydrogen ion concentration to stay within normal limits in the extracellular fluid there must be 1 mEq of carbonic acid for each 20 mEq of bicarbonate. Increases in carbonic acid and decreases in bicarbonate result in acidosis; conversely, increased bicarbonate and decreased carbonic acid result in alkalosis (Brunner and Suddarth, 1975).

Primary bicarbonate deficit (metabolic acidosis or acidemia)

Primary bicarbonate deficit or metabolic acidosis occurs in diarrhea, diabetic ketosis, starvation, infectious diseases, excessive administration of ammonium chloride, salicylate intoxication, overinfusion of normal saline, renal insufficiency, shock, congestive heart failure with tissue anoxia, and with increased serum lactic acid and decreased carbon dioxide.

Signs and symptoms include an increase in the rate and depth of respiration; warm, flushed skin; weakness; disorientation; and coma.

Laboratory findings reveal a urine pH of less than 6.0, plasma bicarbonate level less than 25 mEq/liter, and a plasma pH less than 7.35 (Brunner and Suddarth, 1975; McGaw, 1963).

Primary bicarbonate excess (metabolic alkalosis or alkalemia)

Primary bicarbonate excess or metabolic alkalosis occurs when potassium and chloride are lost through emesis, gastric suctioning; following the excessive use of diuretics, antacids, and steroids; and following the infusion of potassium free solutions.

Signs and symptoms include hypertonicity of muscles, tetany, and depressed respirations.

Laboratory findings reveal a urine pH of 7, plasma bicarbonate greater than 29 mEq/liter, plasma pH greater than 7.45, potassium less than 4 mEq/liter, and a chloride level less than 98 mEq/liter if the alkalosis is caused by hypochloremia (Brunner and Suddarth, 1975; McGaw, 1963).

Primary carbonic acid deficit (respiratory alkalosis or alkalemia)

Primary carbonic acid deficit or respiratory alkalosis is caused by fever, hypoxia, hot weather, encephalitis, salicylate intoxication, hyperventilation, and any condition producing a respiratory depletion of carbon dioxide.

Signs and symptoms include tetany, unconsciousness, and convulsions.

Laboratory findings reveal a urine pH of 7, plasma bicarbonate less than 25 mEq/liter, and plasma pH greater than 7.45 (Brunner and Suddarth, 1975; McGaw, 1963).

Primary carbonic acid excess (respiratory acidosis or acidemia)

Primary carbonic acid excess or respiratory acidosis is caused by chronic pulmonary disease or any factor causing inadequate ventilation.

Table 3. Normal arterial blood gas levels (Shapiro, 1976)

pH	7.35-7.45
Pco_2	35-45 mm Hg
Po_2	80-100 mm Hg
Oxyhemoglobin saturation	Greater than 96%
CO hemoglobin saturation	Variable
Total hemoglobin	12-15 g/100 ml
Plasma bicarbonate	22-28 mEq/liter
Base excess/deficit	±2 mEq/liter
O_2 content	Greater than 16 vol%

Signs and symptoms include a decrease in the rate of respiration, confusion, weakness, cyanosis, and coma.

Laboratory findings reveal a urine pH less than 6, plasma bicarbonate greater than 30 mEq/liter, and plasma pH less than 7.35 (Brunner and Suddarth, 1975; McGaw, 1963).

BLOOD GAS DETERMINATION

Blood gas determination, utilizing arterial blood, is an effective diagnostic tool for determining acidotic and alkalotic states.

Table 3 shows the normal range for arterial blood gases (Shapiro, 1976).

OTHER PROBLEMS RELATED TO IMBALANCES
Plasma–to–interstitial fluid shift (hypovolemia)

Plasma–to–interstitial fluid shift or hypovolemia is a condition related to shock and edema. This shift occurs 24 to 48 hours following severe burns or crushing injuries, perforated peptic ulcers with peritonitis, severe trauma, intestinal obstruction, and venous thrombosis.

Signs and symptoms include pallor, hypotension, tachycardia, cold extremities, and unconsciousness.

Laboratory findings reveal an elevated erythrocyte, hematocrit, and hemoglobin count due to a decreased volume of extracellular fluid (McGaw, 1963).

Interstitial fluid–to–plasma shift (hypervolemia)

Interstitial fluid–to–plasma shift or hypervolemia may occur in the burned patient 3 days following the burn. It is sometimes referred to as remobilization of edema fluid (Brunner and Suddarth, 1975), and it may occur following hemorrhage, fractures, or the administration of osmotic diuretic type fluids such as dextran and plasma.

Signs and symptoms include pallor, air hunger, weakness, and cardiopulmonary overload.

Laboratory findings reveal low erythrocyte, hematocrit, and hemoglobin counts due to the increased volume of circulating extracellular fluid (McGaw, 1963).

Vitamin deficit

Vitamin deficit occurs following starvation or during states that require increased vitamin intake such as injury and infection.

Signs and symptoms depend on which vitamins are depleted (McGaw, 1963).

The most effective diagnostic tools of fluid and electrolyte and acid-base imbalances are laboratory studies, past history, current condition, and physical assessment.

INTRAVENOUS FLUID THERAPY

Intravenous fluids are administered for the purpose of providing nutrition; restoring lost fluids, electrolytes, vitamins, and minerals; maintaining balance during surgical and comatose conditions; and administering medications.

The type and amount of intravenous solution selected is based on the fluid and electrolyte needs of the individual patient.

Monitoring of the patient's response to the therapy is essential and includes assessment and evaluation of both physical and hematologic responses.

The normal average adult (68 kg or 150 lb) requires water, electrolytes, vitamins, carbohydrates, fats, and proteins in the diet.

During each 24-hour period the usual requirements of intake and output of water, sodium, and potassium are as follows:

	Intake	Output
Water	2500-4000 ml	1550-3300 ml (measurable)
Sodium	90-250 mEq	110 mEq
Potassium	80-200 mEq	20-60 mEq

The concentration of the bicarbonate ion is determined by renal function while the concentration of the carbonic acid ion is determined by respiratory function. Increases and decreases in the usual intake and output of substances are dependent on physical activity, individual metabolic rate, and the patient's condition and specific disease.

During states of imbalance the usual requirements may need adjustment in order to increase or decrease the daily intake of fluid, electrolytes, nutrients, and vitamins.

Alterations are made following careful assessment of the patient's condition. Concerns focus on maintenance and replacement.

Maintenance and replacement

Maintenance therapy involves the provision of fluids, electrolytes, nutrients, and vitamins according to the average daily needs of the individual patient. The goal is to maintain a state of equilibrium.

Replacement therapy involves repairing preexisting deficits and providing the components lost due to acute states such as surgery, trauma, burns, shock, vomiting, diarrhea, tubular drainage, wound and burn drainage, and diuresis.

Maintenance therapy provides substances that are routinely required and focuses on ordinary needs, while replacement therapy refers to restoring what is lost prior to therapy and what is acutely lost during therapy. Replacement therapy focuses on extraordinary needs.

Ordinary needs can usually be met by supplying the patient with up to 3000 ml of fluid with added electrolytes, nutrients, and vitamins in a 24-hour period. This dose is generally prescribed at a rate of 1000 ml in each 8-hour period.

Extraordinary needs can be met by replacing what is lost on a volume-to-volume basis. That is to say, for each volume of fluid lost by suction, drainage, or the like, the same volume is replaced. Replacement therapy is over and above maintenance therapy, and as such, it is not unusual to administer fluids to some patients in volumes exceeding 3000 ml in each 24-hour period.

Replacement electrolyte concentration is generally equal to the concentration of electrolytes in the extracellular fluid.

Determining renal function

One of the first steps taken by physicians prior to initiating intravenous fluid therapy is to determine the status of renal function. Potassium excess is often due to renal malfunction, and as such, it is most important to ascertain adequacy of renal function, since potassium excess can produce serious effects.

Adequacy of renal function is determined by reviewing the urine specific gravity, which should be within normal limits (1.003 to 1.030), assessing the patient's urinary output over one or more 24-hour periods, and, if necessary, catheterizing the patient's bladder to determine urine flow.

A traditional method for determining adequacy of urinary function is the Butler method (Brunner and Suddarth, 1975). This involves the administration of a liter of fluid containing 5 mEq sodium, 5 mEq chloride, and 50 g of glucose *or* a liter of fluid containing one part isotonic solution of sodium chloride in 5% dextrose in water. Either solution is administered at a rate of 8 ml/m² body surface per minute for 45 minutes. Should inadequate urine output be due to dehydration, this method will establish flow. The administration of either solution at 2 ml/m² body surface for an additional hour may be necessary.

Should it be determined that there is a renal malfunction, the focus is on correcting the malfunction. There are times when the cause of malfunction is due to a sustained production of ADH invoked by the extra-osmoreceptor mechanism in response to disease (McGaw, 1963).

Once renal function is established, maintenance or replacement therapy or both can be started.

It is difficult to formulate the exact mixture of needed substances; however, when certain principles are followed, a near precise solution can be formulated.

Fluid tonicity

The tonicity of intravenous fluids is measured by comparison with the tonicity of extracellular fluid. Intravenous fluids are categorized as isotonic (having the same tonicity as the extracellular fluid), hypotonic (having a tonicity lower than the extracellular fluid), and hypertonic (having a tonicity greater than the extracellular fluid).

Tonicity is related to the osmolarity of fluids. The tonicity or osmolarity of plasma is 290 mOsm. This is considered isotonic. In order for a solution to be considered hypotonic is must have fewer milliosmols within solution than does an isotonic solution. A significantly fewer number of milliosmols is 50 mOsm less than what is contained in an isotonic solution. In order for a solution to be considered hypertonic it must have more milliosmols within solution than does an isotonic solution. A significantly greater number of milliosmols is 50 mOsm greater than what is contained in an isotonic solution.

Solutions that are isotonic are considered to be compatible with the fluid of the body. Hypotonic solutions, if improperly balanced, can have severe effects when introduced into the vascular system, since osmotic pressure changes cause the solution to move from an area of lesser concentration of solutes to an area of greater concentration. Hence, hypotonic solutions enter red blood cells and cause them to swell and burst, a condition called hemolysis.

Hypertonic solutions, when introduced into the vascular system, have a converse effect. Fluid within the red blood cells by way of osmotic pressure tends to move out of the cells and into the plasma. This causes the red blood cells to shrink, a condition called plasmolysis.

Hypotonic and hypertonic solutions can be balanced with sufficient numbers of electrolytes so that the conditions of hemolysis and plasmolysis can be prevented.

Advantages of infusing electrolyte-balanced hypotonic solutions far outweigh the infusion of solutions containing only dextrose or sodium chloride. Balanced solutions serve to maintain fluid and electrolyte equilibrium.

Hypertonic solutions balanced with electrolytes may or may not include large amounts of dextrose (greater than 10% per liter) and have greater therapeutic usefulness, particularly when administered for the purpose of promoting osmotic diuresis.

Knowledge of the tonicity or osmolarity of a solution aids in determining which solutions are safe to administer subcutaneously, as in hypodermoclysis, and which solutions are safe to administer in conjunction with other substances. As an example, a hypotonic solution such as plain sterile water would be unsafe when administered by infusion; however, then the solution is balanced with the appropriate electrolytes it becomes safe. In addition, plain sterile water would be unsafe when infused because of the destructive effect plain sterile water has on red blood cells.

Dextrose per se elevates the tonicity of solutions, and this is why dextrose 5% in water is considered isotonic. In terms of water and electrolyte balance, dextrose is inconsiderable, since dextrose is metabolized. Plain dextrose and water, as an isotonic solution, eventually intoxicates the patient, since the only remaining substance following metabolism is water. It is therefore necessary to include the essential electrolytes in a balanced formula, since electrolytes are not metabolized as such.

Normal saline, or 0.9% saline solution, or physiologic saline solution is also considered unsafe when administered over a relatively short period of time. The concentration of sodium and chloride is 154 mEq/liter of each, and the milliosmolar level is in keeping with isotonicity. However, there is no potassium or magnesium present. The results include a sodium and chloride excess and a potassium and magnesium deficit.

THERAPIES
Maintenance

During *maintenance therapy* a balanced hypotonic electrolyte solution with the addition of 5% dextrose for calories is ideal. This balanced solution contains the following cations and anions per liter (Abbott, 1969):

Cations		Anions	
Sodium	40 mEq/liter	Chloride	40 mEq/liter
Potassium	13 mEq/liter	Acetate	16 mEq/liter
Magnesium	3 mEq/liter		
TOTAL	56 mEq/liter	TOTAL	56 mEq/liter

During each 24-hour period, 3000 ml of the balanced hypotonic electrolyte solution should be administered, 1000 ml over each 8-hour period.

The hypotonicity of the electrolytes permits the kidneys to retain or excrete water while the dextrose supplies calories and prevents hemolysis of the red blood cells.

Replacement

Ideally, replacement therapy solutions should contain ions in the same composition as that of the plasma and interstitial fluid. This would categorize this type of solution as a balanced isotonic multiple electrolyte solution. Dextrose may or may not be included, depending on the caloric needs of the patient. It should be emphasized that sodium depletion, especially in gastrointestinal disorders, results in potassium depletion. Therefore the potassium deficit occurring within the intracellular fluid should be replaced. The loss of hydrochloric acid by way of gastric suction leads to a chloride deficit. This is called hypochloremic alkalosis. The loss of intestinal secretions produces metabolic acidosis, since these secretions are highly alkaline (Abbott, 1969).

A balanced isotonic multiple electrolyte solution would include the following cations and anions with or without 5% dextrose/liter:

Cations		Anions	
Sodium	140 mEq/liter	Chloride	98 mEq/liter
Potassium	5 mEq/liter	Acetate	27 mEq/liter
Magnesium	3 mEq/liter	Gluconate	23 mEq/liter
TOTAL	148 mEq/liter	TOTAL	148 mEq/liter

This solution has an average pH of 6.2. Most intravenous solutions have an acid pH. Acid pH solutions are more stable and are better able to withstand the effects of bacterial overgrowth.

A disadvantage of acid pH solutions is the patient's predisposition to chemical phlebitis.

Therapies for special needs
SURGICAL PATIENT

Patients having elective surgery with no previous deficit and no concurrent losses will require the replacement formula during the surgical procedure.

Should the patient be dehydrated prior to surgery, 1 to 2 liters of the replacement formula are required.

During the first 24 hours following the surgical procedure, a combination of the replacement and maintenance formula will be necessary. Usually no more than 3000 ml of the two will be required.

During the second 24 hours following surgery and the days that follow, and until the patient can be maintained by oral intake, an infusion of two-thirds maintenance formula and one-third replacement formula with added 5% dextrose and 20 mEq potassium chloride will be necessary. Doses of multivitamins may be added to every other liter or to at least 1 liter during each 24-hour period (Baxter, 1972).

Patients having special surgery will require replacement of previous deficits and concurrent losses (Baxter, 1972). The focus is on supplying maintenance needs as well as replacement needs on a volume-to-volume basis.

DIABETIC ACIDOSIS

During diabetic acidosis the aim is to correct deficits and supply insulin. The blood is acid, ketone bodies are present, the blood sugar is elevated, and there is a state of hyperosmolality. The patient is losing large amounts of water, sodium, potassium, and some anions due to a state of osmotic diuresis (Baxter, 1972).

The effectiveness of insulin is altered when the pH is not normal and during states of altered renal function. In order that acid metabolites be excreted and the formation of ammonia be resumed, a balance must be restored.

The key substances in this diabetic acidotic state are insulin, water, sodium, potassium, and carbohydrates.

The ideal treatment is the administration of insulin, nasogastric suction to remove the very acidotic secretions, and the administration of the replacement formula at a rate of 240 to 360 ml/hour. To effect rehydration and volume-to-volume replacement, 20 mEq potassium chloride is usually added to this formula (Baxter, 1972).

Urine sugar and acetone levels, arterial blood gases, venous glucose, acetone, sodium, potassium, and urea levels should be determined and used as guides to further therapy.

Sodium bicarbonate is administered until the blood pH is greater than 7.2. The usual dosage is 0.5 mEq sodium bicarbonate per kilogram of body weight administered over a 10- to 15-minute period. After an initial dose, the blood pH should be determined, and if necessary, additional doses of sodium bicarbonate are administered at 30-minute intervals until such time as the blood pH level is 7.2 or slightly higher.

At this point no more sodium bicarbonate is administered even if the base deficit carbon dioxide content is still significantly low (Baxter, 1972).

Only when the blood pH is above 7.2 will insulin be effective. Sodium bicarbonate reduces the insulin requirements. As an example, with sufficient sodium bicarbonate, a dosage of 150 units of insulin may be adequate, whereas with insufficient sodium bicarbonate, a dosage of 300 to 400 units of insulin may be necessary (Baxter, 1972).

Continuation of hydration can be accomplished by the administration of the maintenance therapy formula with the addition of 20 to 40 mEq of potassium chloride. In severe diabetic acidosis up to 100 mEq/liter of potassium chloride may be required during the first hours of therapy (Baxter, 1972). Extreme caution should be taken when such high dosages of potassium chloride are used.

SHOCK

During states of shock with accompanying hypotension, poor tissue perfusion caused by microcirculatory stasis and lowered blood volume caused by a shift of fluid from the extracellular to intracellular compartments, there is decreased effectiveness of the circulating blood volume.

The aim of therapy during shock is to correct the hypovolemic state. Adequate tissue perfusion depends on plasma volume, and therefore perfusion will be poor with a hematocrit count exceeding 45%. Optimum oxygen carrying capacity of hemoglobin occurs when the hematocrit count is at 30% to 35% because the blood viscosity is lower. High blood viscosity causes sludging or cell aggregation with accompanying impairment of circulation at the cellular level (Baxter, 1972).

The amount of replacement fluid depends on the patient's condition and the type of shock. Cardiogenic versus noncardiogenic shock should be differentiated (Baxter, 1972).

Central venous pressure monitoring is a guide to determining adequacy of fluid replacement (Baxter, 1972).

Restoration of the circulating volume of fluid can be accomplished with low molecular dextran solutions. This solution expands the plasma and enhances microcirculation. In addition, there is an osmotic movement of interstitial fluid into the vascular channels with accompanying improvement of peripheral blood flow, improved venous return, and increased cardiac output (Baxter, 1972).

The initial dosage of low molecular dextran should not exceed 20 ml/kg of body weight during the first 24 hours of therapy and 10 ml/kg of body weight thereafter. Larger doses may prolong bleeding time and increase blood losses. Dextran may interfere with blood matching and falsely elevate blood sugar, bilirubin, and total protein.

Dextran should not be used in the presence of marked thrombocytopenia, hypofibrinogenemia, or renal diseases with severe oliguria or anuria (Baxter, 1972).

Extracellular fluid replacement can be accomplished by adding the replacement formula to this regimen.

Acidosis can be corrected with the addition of sodium bicarbonate or tromethamine. Dosage is determined by laboratory findings.

Other treatment during shock includes administration of oxygen, antihypotensive medications, calcium following multiple transfusions, sodium bicarbonate in a dose of 50 mEq for each three units of whole blood administered, and prevention of heat loss by the application of blankets. Nonactive heating methods should be used. It is preferable to administer all required medications by way of the intravenous route, since tissue perfusion is poor at this time.

MANNITOL (OSMITROL) THERAPY

Mannitol (Osmitrol) is a sugar alcohol solution that acts as an osmotic diuretic. It is used to reduce intracranial pressure and intraocular pressure, to promote excretion of toxins following drug overdose, to reduce edema and ascites, and to test kidney function.

Electrolyte depletion may occur following the administration of mannitol (Gahart, 1977).

BURN THERAPY

The initial response to severe burns is shock caused by a shift of the extracellular fluid from the plasma to the interstitial space. This is aggravated by an outpouring of fluid into the burned area. This occurs apart from the fluid that is also lost from the denuded burned areas. With burns involving 25% of the body surface, the volume of edema fluid may equal 50% of the total volume of extracellular fluid. The main component of the extracellular fluid shifting is water, and, as such, the plasma becomes concentrated, causing dehydration with resulting microcirculatory stasis and acidosis. Renal damage is a threat due to a release of hemoglobin, which occurs from the destruction of red blood cells, which break down 2 to 3 days following the burn (Baxter, 1972).

Pulmonary damage from smoke and flame inhalation may occur. This, coupled with capillary malfunction, can alter bicarbonate regulation.

Resorption of large amounts of edema fluid begins on the second or third day, and therefore too much initial fluid therapy predisposes the patient to pulmonary edema.

Large quantities of sodium shift to the burned areas, and intracellular potassium is exchanged for the sodium. With diuresis accompanying the resorption of edema fluid, more sodium is lost. The patient may be in a state of negative sodium balance for weeks following burns.

With the administration of plasma, protein levels may be elevated during the early stages; however, the patient loses more protein than is assimilated until the burns are healed (Baxter, 1972).

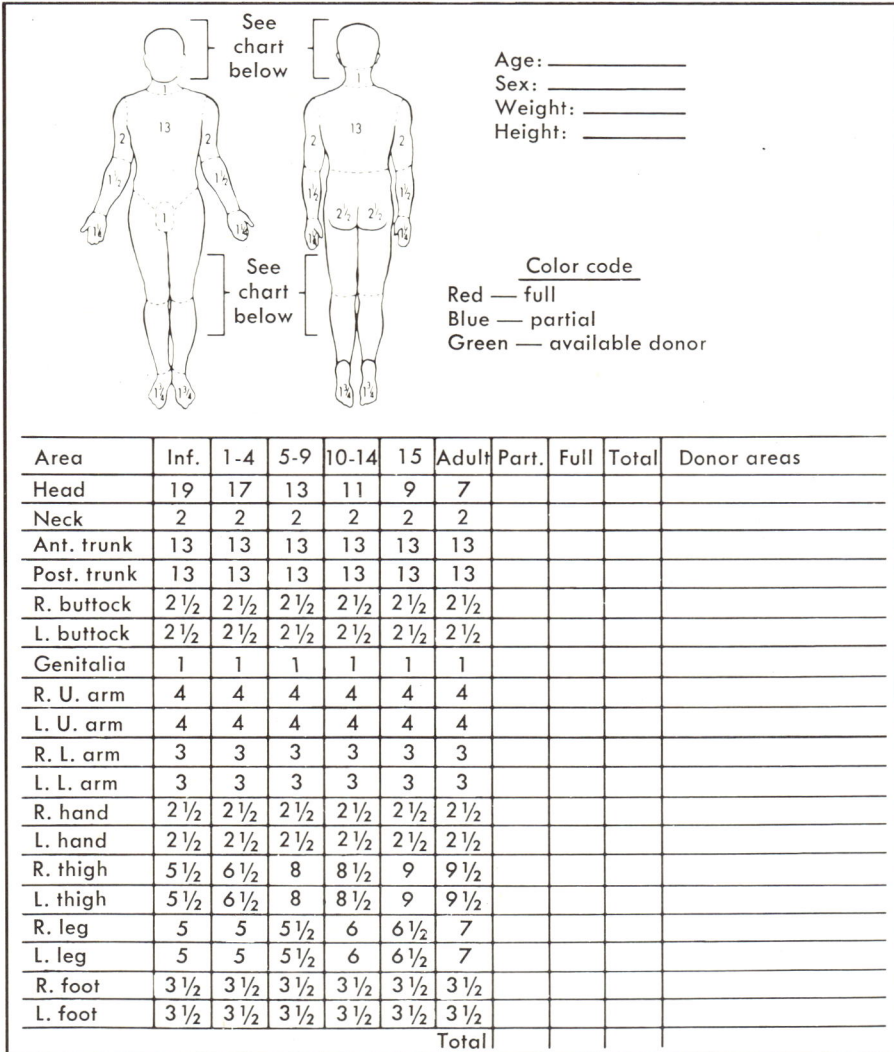

Area	Inf.	1-4	5-9	10-14	15	Adult	Part.	Full	Total	Donor areas
Head	19	17	13	11	9	7				
Neck	2	2	2	2	2	2				
Ant. trunk	13	13	13	13	13	13				
Post. trunk	13	13	13	13	13	13				
R. buttock	2½	2½	2½	2½	2½	2½				
L. buttock	2½	2½	2½	2½	2½	2½				
Genitalia	1	1	1	1	1	1				
R. U. arm	4	4	4	4	4	4				
L. U. arm	4	4	4	4	4	4				
R. L. arm	3	3	3	3	3	3				
L. L. arm	3	3	3	3	3	3				
R. hand	2½	2½	2½	2½	2½	2½				
L. hand	2½	2½	2½	2½	2½	2½				
R. thigh	5½	6½	8	8½	9	9½				
L. thigh	5½	6½	8	8½	9	9½				
R. leg	5	5	5½	6	6½	7				
L. leg	5	5	5½	6	6½	7				
R. foot	3½	3½	3½	3½	3½	3½				
L. foot	3½	3½	3½	3½	3½	3½				
						Total				

Fig. 5-3. Estimation of percentage of burned areas. (From Jacoby, F. G.: Nursing care of the patient with burns, ed. 2, St. Louis, 1976, The C. V. Mosby Co.)

Fluid and electrolyte therapy must be carefully monitored. Close monitoring of urine volume, specific gravity, and gastric drainage is also necessary.

Fig. 5-3 shows a chart that is useful in estimating the percentage of burned areas.

During the first 24 hours, therapy for severe second- and third-degree burns exceeding 15% of body surface includes one-half of the total daily required fluids and electrolytes administered during the first 8-hour period followed by one-fourth of the total daily required fluids and electrolytes over the second and third 8-hour periods.

For burns exceeding 15% of the body surface, a replacement of fluids in the amount of 10% of the patient's body weight is indicated. One-fourth of this replacement should include sodium bicarbonate and three-fourths should be in the form of the replacement formula. The amount of sodium bicarbonate administered is determined by serum pH levels. Total fluid replacement should not exceed 150 ml/kg of body weight.

During the second 24-hour period, similar formulas are used as in the first 24-hour period; however, one-half the amount will be required.

After this initial phase, a maintenance formula may be used. Since the caloric and protein requirements are great, total parenteral nutrition solutions are generally employed (Baxter, 1972).

OTHER INTRAVENOUS SOLUTIONS

Other intravenous solutions employed during IV therapy are carbohydrate in water solutions, carbohydrate in sodium chloride solutions, isotonic sodium chloride solutions, potassium solutions, vitamin solutions, protein hydrolysate solutions, and alcohol solutions. Fructose may be utilized instead of dextrose, since fructose is more rapidly metabolized and more rapidly converted to glycogen (Baxter, 1972).

Used in proper combination, these solutions are adequate for at least 80% of the patients requiring intravenous therapy.

A list of terminology associated with solutions can be found in the Appendix.

References

Abbott Laboratories: Fluid and electrolytes, North Chicago, Ill., 1969, Abbott Laboratories.

Baxter Laboratories: The fundamentals of body water and electrolytes, Deerfield, Ill., Oct. 1972.

Brunner, L., and Suddarth, D.: Textbook of medical-surgical nursing, ed. 3, New York, 1975, J. B. Lippincott Co.

Gahart, B.: Intravenous medications: a handbook for nurses and other allied health personnel, ed. 2, St. Louis, 1977, The C. V. Mosby Co.

Guyton, A.: Textbook of medical physiology, ed. 5, Philadelphia, 1976, W. B. Saunders Co.

Johnson, W., et al.: Biology, ed. 4, New York, 1972, Holt, Rinehart & Winston.

Kabat, H., and Price, E.: Intravenous therapy in-service training series, clinical seminar no. 2, intravenous incompatibility, 1971.

McGaw Laboratories: Guide to parenteral fluid therapy, Glendale, Calif., 1963.

Plumer, A.: Principles and practice of intravenous therapy, ed. 2, Boston, 1975, Little, Brown & Co.

Shapiro, B.: Clinical application of blood gases, Chicago, 1976, Yearbook Medical Publishers.

Thomas, C., editor: Taber's cyclopedic medical dictionary, ed. 13, Philadelphia, 1977, F. A. Davis Co.

Chapter 6

Complications of intravenous therapy

The complications of intravenous therapy are varied and are categorized as local, systemic, and mechanical.

Immediate recognition of impending problems by continuously observing the patient's responses to all aspects of intravenous therapy is an effective method of preventing complications.

Other methods used for preventing IV-related complications include employing safe practices, following agency policies and procedures, using sufficient numbers of properly trained personnel, and adhering to infection control guidelines (Francke, 1973).

This chapter serves to review IV-related complications by category. Included in the review are definitions, methods of identification, prevention, and nursing implications.

LOCAL COMPLICATIONS

Local complications are those that occur in and around the venipuncture site. Local complications include extravasation and infiltration; hematoma; sclerosis; and chemical, mechanical, and septic reactions.

Extravasation and infiltration

Extravasation, which is a leaking of fluid into the tissues around the IV site, occurs when the vein wall is punctured secondarily to the initial penetration or when the fluid is flowing into the surrounding tissue rather than into the vein. The latter occurs when the needle or cannula inadvertently slips out of the vein.

Infiltration is the accumulation of extravasating fluid. Infiltration causes the tissues to become edematous, giving the area involved a characteristic puffy appearance. The skin appears white in color and it may feel hard and cool to touch. The patient may feel pain and burning. Necrosis and sloughing may occur following infiltration of irritating solutions.

Methods used to evaluate whether a needle or cannula is in the vein include checking for backflow of blood into the IV tubing by pinching its flash chamber or by lowering the fluid container below the level of the infusion site. Altered pressures within the vein with a resulting collapse of the vein or cannula may prevent blood from backflowing; therefore the aforementioned tests are not absolute.

Careful insertion of the needle or cannula, using recommended taping techniques, and avoiding the application of undue pressure to the infusion site as occurs during lifting and moving, blood pressure monitoring, and restraining, aid in preventing infiltration.

Should infiltration occur, discontinue the infusion and restart it in the opposite extremity or in the same extremity proximal to the infiltrated area.

Independent nursing action to treat infiltration includes elevation of the affected part to promote venous drainage and the application of warm, moist compresses to improve circulation.

In the case of infiltration of irritating drugs, it may become necessary to inject specific antidotes into the site of infiltration. For example, reserpine is injected directly into the infiltrated site in an effort to counteract the necrotizing effects of levarterenol bitartrate. The physician is responsible for such treatment.

Hematoma

A hematoma may develop following an unsuccessful attempt at venipuncture or when a blood transfusion infiltrates. A hematoma appears as a raised ecchymosed area. Should a hematoma develop, nursing action includes removal of the needle or cannula, application of pressure, and application of cold compresses.

Phlebitis, thrombophlebitis, phlebothrombosis, and sclerosis

Phlebitis, thrombophlebitis, phlebothrombosis, and sclerosis occur as a result of vein irritation and inflammation with or without clot formation. Abscesses may form later.

Phlebitis is inflammation of a vein. It is characterized by pain, tenderness, a red skin discoloration, and edema of the vein and surrounding tissues.

Thrombophlebitis is inflammation of a vein with clot formation. It is characterized by pain and inflammation along the course of the vein. In addition, the vein may become hard, tortuous, and tender. Fever, malaise, and leukocytosis may occur, and there is a danger of embolism (Plumer, 1975).

Phlebothrombosis is the formation of a clot without marked vein inflammation (Brunner and Suddarth, 1975). The danger of embolism is present; some authorities feel that phlebothrombosis is a major source of pulmonary emboli. Phlebothrombosis usually occurs in veins of the lower extremities.

Sclerosis is the thickening and hardening (induration) of the layers of a vein. A clot may form, eventually develop into connective tissue, and cause sclerosis. Formation of fibrous tissue later results in permanent occlusion of the vein. Highly concentrated dextrose solutions, when injected into small veins, produce sclerosis.

Chemical, mechanical, and septic reactions

Chemical, mechanical, and septic reactions cause phlebitis, thrombophlebitis, phlebothrombosis, and sclerosis.

Chemical reactions are most commonly due to the use of acid, alcohol, or highly hypertonic solutions, and to the body's reaction to foreign substances. Avoid chemical reactions by administering irritating substances only after adequate dilution. In addition, it is advisable to use solutions that have a neutral or near neutral pH. Inject sclerosing agents into large veins with copious blood flow. For example, administer dextrose solutions that exceed a concentration of 10% into the subclavian vein.

Avoid using small veins when administering alcohol and acid solutions.

Avoid mechanical reactions by selecting, using, and adequately immobilizing appropriate needles and cannulae. Use stainless steel needles or hypoallergenic cannulae, since some patients are allergic to certain plastics. To immobilize the needle or cannula, tape the set in such a fashion as to prevent excessive (to-and-fro) movement.

Septic reactions are related to the patient's disease, age, sex, the use of filters, duration of therapy, and the degree to which infection control is practiced.

Nursing action related to chemical, mechanical, and septic reactions includes sound infection control practices, filtering of particulate matter, site rotation, avoiding the use of small veins for administering alcohol, acid, and very hypertonic solutions, adequate taping techniques, and the assessment of all signs and symptoms related to this group of complications. It is necessary to implement appropriate preventive and supportive techniques such as frequent inspection of the venipuncture site and observation for pain, redness, and edema along the course of the vein. At the first sign of a complication, discontinue the infusion and restart at another site if the therapy is to be continued. Consult the physician and document all action.

SYSTEMIC COMPLICATIONS

Systemic complications occur apart from local complications and include pyrogenic reactions such as septicemia and bacteremia; pulmonary embolism; air embolism; catheter embolism; pulmonary edema; speed shock; nerve damage; pneumothorax; hydrothorax; and hemothorax.

Recognition of systemic complications is based on careful observation of specific signs and symptoms such as chills, fever, headache, backache, nausea, vomiting, shortness of breath, cyanosis, syncope, paralysis, and shocklike states.

Pyrogenic reactions

Pyrogenic reactions are generalized infections resulting from the use of contaminated equipment or solutions. Pyrogenic reactions include septicemia and bacteremia. Employing infection control practices such as using sterile equipment and sterile technique in initiating venipuncture and during site care, avoiding contamination of solutions, especially those that have high concentrations of dextrose, changing containers and tubings every 24 hours, and rotating sites every 72 hours serve to prevent pyrogenic reactions.

Pulmonary embolism

Pulmonary embolism denotes obstruction of the pulmonary artery or its large branches by thrombi originating in peripheral veins. Sudden death may follow pulmonary embolism.

Prevention of pulmonary embolism includes discontinuing infusions at the first sign of phlebitis, avoiding irrigation of clotted infusions, and avoiding the use of veins of the lower extremities.

Air embolism

Any given amount of air may inadvertently enter the vascular system, reach the heart, and produce cardiac arrest.

Animal experiments indicate that up to 500 to 1000 ml of air administered intravenously has been tolerated. The injected air is filtered out of the vascular system by way of the pulmonary system unless there is a septal defect within the heart or the presence of a shunt. Consideration is given to the pressure and rate at which the air is infused.

In humans the administration of up to 10 ml of air intravascularly can have serious, if not fatal, effects. Safe practice indicates the avoidance of all air; however, small bubbles of air may be tolerated by most patients.

Hypotension, cyanosis, heart murmur, tachycardia, syncope, vascular collapse, and loss of consciousness are signs and symptoms of air embolism. The risk of air embolism is greater in large veins where negative pressure may actually pull air into the vascular system. With any shunt the air goes directly to the brain. It may take up to 20 minutes for the signs and symptoms of air embolism to become evident. Air embolism is considered an emergency situation.

Treatment includes immediately turning the patient on his left side in a Trendelenburg position in order to displace the air away from the outflow tract of the right ventricle (McGill, 1973). Improvement in the patient's condition is soon evident if the signs and symptoms are related to air embolism.

Air embolism can be prevented by using closed-system infusion sets and by avoiding the introduction of air into the vascular system. Other methods for preventing air from entering the system and for removal of air from the system include ascertaining that the tubing drip chamber is one-half full of fluid at all times, removing all air from tubings prior to connecting them to the patient, displacing air that has inadvertently entered the tubing by rolling the infusion tubing onto a pen or pencil distal to the air and the drip chamber until the air is displaced into the drip chamber, inserting a needle with syringe into the flash chamber or side arm of the tubing set and withdrawing the air, inserting a small guage needle into the flash chamber or side arm of the tubing in order to shunt the air out of the tubing, clamping the system shut when changing containers and tubings, and securing all tubing junctions.

Catheter embolism

Catheter embolism occurs when a portion of a plastic cannula inadvertently breaks off and flows into the vascular system. Catheter breaks occur following repeated to-and-fro movement and when cannulae are severed by needle stylets during insertion. Prevention of catheter embolism includes using recommended taping techniques, avoiding the rethreading of stylets into cannulae once cannula threading begins, and by using needle protectors on all in-the-needle catheters.

If not retrieved, lost catheters may lodge in a peripheral vein or migrate to the heart or lungs. Catheter fragments may puncture the wall of a large vein or the heart, causing hemorrhage and cardiac tamponade, which results in a surgical emergency (Abbott, 1972). X-ray verification of catheter placement and location is usually possible since most are radiopaque.

Retrieval of catheter fragments lodged in peripheral veins is possible by use of the percutaneous catheter snare technique (Abbott, 1972), in which a small gauge catheter, through which a wire loop is inserted, captures and retrieves the lost fragment.

Tourniqueting extremities prior to discontinuing peripheral plastic cannulae may serve to prevent catheter embolism. The tourniquet is placed proximal to the tip of the catheter. Immediately following removal of the catheter and verification of its intactness, the tourniquet is removed and pressure is applied to the venipuncture site.

Pulmonary edema

Pulmonary edema generally follows circulatory overload. Pulmonary edema can be prevented through careful adherence to administering fluids at the prescribed rate. Signs and symptoms of pulmonary edema include headache, hypertension, coughing, and dyspnea. Pulmonary edema occurs most often in geriatric patients and patient with decreased cardiac output.

During the acute phase of pulmonary edema the infusion should be slowed to a keep-open rate, the patient placed in a high Fowler's position, and the physician notified.

Steps toward preventing pulmonary edema include monitoring infusion flow rates every 30 to 60 minutes. Flooding of patients with excessive infusion fluid appears to occur most often during shift changes; therefore monitoring of flow rates is to be delegated to one who is uninvolved with the many duties incurred during shift changes.

Speed shock

Speed shock occurs when solutions and medications are rapidly administered into the vascular system. Plasma concentrations reach toxic proportions. Signs and symptoms of speed shock include shock, syncope, and cardiac arrest. Speed shock can be prevented by using controlled-volume infusion sets and controllers (Fig. 6-1).

IV controllers give added protection by preventing large quantities of fluid from being accidentally infused.

Using an extra clamp on the IV tubing ensures greater safety should the primary clamp accidentally release.

Upon initiating the infusion, ensure that the solution is flowing freely prior to adjusting the rate. Movement of the needle in which the aperture is partially obstructed by the wall of the vein could cause an increase in the flow, contributing to the dangers of speed shock.

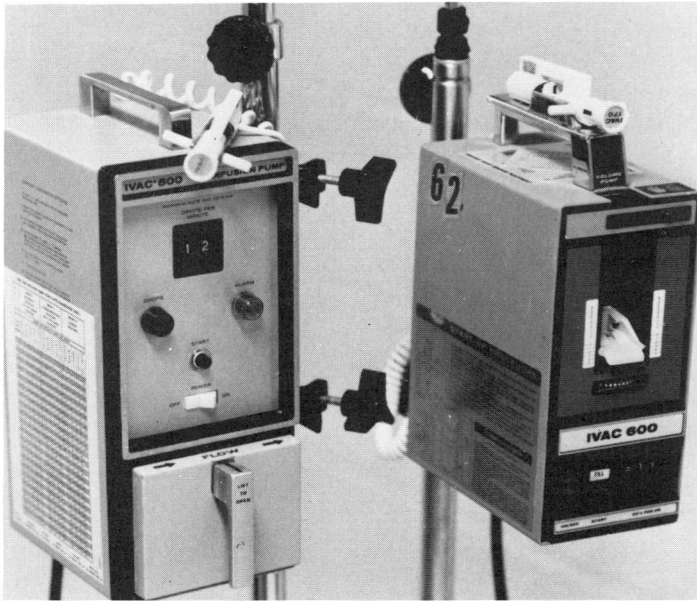

Fig. 6-1. IV controllers aid in prevention of speed shock. (Courtesy Alton Ochsner Medical Foundation, New Orleans.)

Nerve damage

Nerve damage occurs when needles or cannulae accidentally injure underlying nerves near or at the site of venipuncture, and when parts are improperly immobilized with tape and hand or arm boards.

Brachial plexus palsy occurs when the lateral zone lying anterior to the first rib is punctured during subclavian venipuncture. Signs and symptoms of brachial plexus palsy include tingling of the fingers, pain radiating down the arm, and paralysis of the arm.

Pneumothorax, hydrothorax, and hemothorax

Pneumothorax, hydrothorax, and hemothorax may occur following subclavian venipuncture. The terminology implies air, water, and blood entering the pleural cavity due to puncture of the inferior wall of the subclavian vein and the pleura. It is because of pneumothorax, hydrothorax, and hemothorax that x-ray verification of subclavian catheter placement is vital.

MECHANICAL COMPLICATIONS

Mechanical complications occur as a result of changes in the position of the needle in the vein, height of the solution, amount of solution remaining in the container, venospasm, position of the patient, kinked tubes, disconnected tubes, plugged air vents, and plugged needles and cannulae.

Control of mechanical failures centers around observation and assessment of adequate functioning of the entire system.

Safety measures include keeping the patient's call bell, bedside stand, and water, if allowed, within easy reach, and assisting the patient with feeding as necessary.

During ambulation, trips to other departments, and on returning to bed, the rate of flow is evaluated.

References

Abbott Laboratories: Venipuncture and venous cannulation, North Chicago, Ill., 1971, Abbott Laboratories.

Brunner, L., and Suddarth, D.: Textbook of medical-surgical nursing, ed. 2, Philadelphia, 1975, J. B. Lippincott Co.

Francke, D.: Handbook of IV additive review, Drug intelligence publication, Hamilton, Ill., 1973, The Hamilton Press.

McGill, D.: Giving IV push, Nursing 73, June 1973.

Plumer, A.: Principles and practice of intravenous therapy, ed. 2, Boston, 1975, Little, Brown & Co.

Chapter 7

Total parenteral nutrition

Total parenteral nutrition (TPN) implies the administration, by needle, of all nutrients required by the body.

Parenteral hyperalimentation implies the administration of nutrients required by the body in excess of what is normally required. Traditional hyperalimentation formulas supply all of the required nutrients except fat.

The terminology, total parenteral nutrition (TPN), although confusing, since the prefix "hyper" is not included, apparently means the administration of all that is required to meet the specific nutritional needs of the individual patient.

The TPN formula includes the nutrients needed during ordinary circumstances plus those nutrients needed during extraordinary circumstances. The terminology, total parenteral nutrition (TPN), will be used in this text.

The purpose of TPN is to achieve or maintain tissue synthesis, positive nitrogen balance, and anabolism (Beland and Passos, 1975).

TPN, excluding intralipid therapy, has been successfully administered to humans since the early 1960s. Credit for success is given to Dr. S. J. Dudrick and his colleagues, Drs. D. W. Wilmore, H. M. Vars, and J. E. Rhoads.

The TPN formula consists of protein hydrolysate or crystalline amino acids in a concentration of 5%, carbohydrates in a concentration of 25% or more, water, 5% electrolytes, vitamins, trace elements, and insulin, either added to the formula or given separately every 4 to 6 hours as needed. The specific formula is determined by the needs of the patient (Beland and Passos, 1975).

Previous attempts at using protein and highly concentrated dextrose solutions were made during the 1940s; however, the failure rate was great because these solutions were usually administered through peripheral veins. Not until it was realized that solutions of this type could be administered by way of great veins such as the subclavian and internal or external jugular vein was success realized.

Dextrose in concentrations exceeding 10% has a sclerosing effect on veins, and by using the larger veins, adequate and rapid dilution of the dextrose by the blood is possible. This prevents the common and painful phlebotic and sclerotic effects that were seen in the early days of therapy.

Intralipid therapy (fat emulsion therapy) or the administration of fat by the intravenous route can be accomplished by administering this solution concurrent to TPN or alone. The high caloric value of fat and its advantages in parenteral nutrition have been recognized for many years.

Administration of fat solutions in the United States was first attempted in the early 1950s. A cottonseed oil preparation was used at that time. It failed because of the usually fatal complication of fat embolism.

Intralipid therapy was first successfully administered to humans in Sweden during the early 1960s. During that time a Swedish investigator discovered an improved emulsifier, which is known as 10% intravenous fat emulsion (10% intralipid by Cutter Laboratories).

Ten percent intralipid fat emulsion is comprised of 10% soybean oil, 1.2% egg yolk phospholipid, 2.25% glycerine, and pyrogen-free water. This preparation has been widely used in Europe and has been under clinical investigation in the United States.

Ten percent intralipid fat emulsion has been shown to be effective with a low incidence of side effects and seldom causes the once feared side effects associated with cottonseed oil preparations. Intralipid therapy was approved for use in the United States by the Food and Drug Administration in 1974.

RATIONALE FOR USE

During certain disease processes and following certain surgical procedures, it may be impossible for a patient to take any form of or an adequate amount of oral nutrition. This problem may persist for several days or for as long as 4 to 6 weeks. These conditions are listed as esophageal atresia, intestinal obstruction, inflammatory bowel diseases such as regional enteritis and chronic ulcerative colitis, gastrointestinal fistulae, pyloric stenosis, massive bowel resection, short bowel syndrome, metastatic carcinoma with radiation where nausea, vomiting, and anorexia occurs. Major burns, anorexia nervosa, acute and chronic pancreatitis, chronic uncontrolled diarrhea and severe intractable malabsorption syndrome, hypermetabolic states stemming from multiple injuries, serious infections such as peritonitis, acute hepatic failure, fractures, trauma, emotional stress, gastric and intestinal carcinoma, decubitus ulcers, chronic debilitating conditions, and any disease of the gastrointestinal tract where oral feedings are impossible or ill advised.

It is virtually impossible to supply the extraordinary caloric and other nutritional needs of patients during the aforementioned conditions with traditional intravenous therapy. Without adequate replacement of vital nutrients, the patient develops a condition described by Kaminski (1976) as protein calorie malnutrition.

This malnutrition is characterized by muscle wasting, decubitus and stress ulcer formation, indolent wounds forming poor granulation tissue, weight loss in excess of 10% of the preillness weight, low serum albumin and total protein, poor leukocyte function, and lowered resistance to infection.

The normal adult at rest requires approximately 400 calories during each 24-hour period in order to preserve body protein. Postoperatively the same adult would require approximately 1500 calories to preserve body protein. Should the patient develop fever or other complications, or have certain diseases as previously mentioned, he or she may require from 2000 to 10,000 calories during each 24-hour period. This large amount required lessens as the patient progresses toward a state of wellness.

During these chronic and ultradebilitating diseases the patient suffers from malnutrition. His stores of protein are depleted. As a result a metabolic imbalance, specifically, a negative nitrogen balance, develops. He is in a state of catabolism. This is due to a response to stress where the hypothalamus is stimulated. The sympathetic nervous system is triggered, causing the pancreas to decrease its insulin output and increase its glucagon production. This is carried out by action from the anti-insulin hormone. An increase in epinephrine is produced by the adrenal glands, causing a potentiating effect to occur by norepinephrine on the glucoregulating hormone. Glucagon, the anti-insulin hormone, causes proteolysis, gluconeogenesis, lipolysis, ketogenesis, and glycogenolysis to occur. The response results in malabsorption or no absorption of nutrients by the cells (Kaminski, 1976).

In addition, excessive cortisol is secreted by the adrenal cortex. This too effects proteolysis within the cells. The growth hormone stimulates catabolism of glycogen and fat during this period.

The TPN solution can promote anabolism even in the presence of the disease process.

A hyperinsulinemic state allows protein (amino acids) to enter the cells. The growth hormone allows for protein production. Glycolysis increases the production of adenosine triphosphate (ATP), and enzymes restore glycogen in the liver and muscles. Fatty acids, triglycerides, and glucose enter the cells and convert into fat. TPN also provides the needed electrolytes and nutrients for the cells.

Highly concentrated dextrose solutions, without amino acids, can suppress the growth hormone and produce scurvy, which in turn delays wound healing.

During the state of hyperinsulinemia and hypogluconemia, the hepatic enzyme systems are suppressed, causing a suppression in the conversion of amino acids to glucose and urea.

To convert the patient from a catabolic to anabolic state the nitrogen balance during each 24-hour period should be +4 to +6 g. Once converted into an anabolic state, the positive nitrogen balance may be 12 to 20 g or more during each 24-hour period.

Insulin shock is possible, since the TPN solution can decrease the production of the anti-insulin hormone.

TPN SOLUTION

In order to prevent overloading the patient with excessive amounts of water, highly concentrated dextrose solutions are used to prepare TPN solutions.

A liter of 5% dextrose in water contains 50 g of carbohydrate, which supplies 200 calories. In order to provide 2,000 to 10,000 calories, a more concentrated solution of dextrose is necessary. A liter of 20% dextrose contains 200 g of carbohydrate, which supplies 800 calories, and a liter of 50% dextrose in water contains 500 g of carbohydrate and 2,000 calories.

Although 50% solutions of dextrose in water are used to prepare TPN solutions, the end solution will contain a concentration of approximately 20% to 25% dextrose, since it is diluted with other fluids. Fructose solutions, which can be used without insulin, are sometimes employed (Beland and Passos, 1975).

Since hypertonic solutions cause osmotic diuresis and glycosuria, it is advisable to begin TPN administration at a slow rate. Approximately 60 ml administered during the first hour and no more than 125 ml/hour thereafter can prevent the occurrence of these complications.

Utilization of large, central veins will prevent thrombophlebitis and sclerosis because adequate dilution of the solution can be obtained. When the therapy is discontinued, it is advisable to taper the patient off in order to prevent hypoglycemia and other complications.

Hypoglycemia or hyperglycemia can occur when solutions of high dextrose concentrations are administered at uneven rates of flow. This necessitates keeping the rate of flow constant and avoiding "catching up" of solutions that have inadvertently lagged behind. Checking the rate of flow every 30 to 60 minutes and using intravenous controllers minimizes this problem.

The patient's urine should be checked for sugar and acetone every 4 to 6 hours, and additional regular insulin should be administered as necessary using the sliding scale method.

Ethyl alcohol, which contains 7 calories per gram, can be used as an additional source of energy. Some complications associated with the use of ethyl alcohol include inebriation and venous pain. Ethyl alcohol is contraindicated in patients with liver disease.

Protein in the form of protein hydrolysate or crystalline amino acids is administered according to the patient's needs. The amount needed is calculated from known nitrogen loss. The protein administered includes all of the essential amino acids and some or all of the nonessential amino acids. The presence of all amino acids (essential and nonessential) improves the utilization of amino acids by the body.

The synthetic amino acids (crystalline amino acids, FreAmine) seem to be more satisfactory in achieving nitrogen balance.

The protein hydrolysates (Amigen, Aminosol, and Hyprotigen) are acid or enzymatic digests of casein, protein, lactalbumin, blood fibrin, or other suitable protein. These preparations differ in amino acid and electrolyte content (Smith, Kline, and French, 1975).

The amount of protein in a TPN solution is determined by the nitrogen-to-calorie ratio. To assure complete utilization, the ratio should be 1 g nitrogen to 150 calories. 4.5 g nitrogen equals 28 g protein.

Amino acids, when administered alone, convert to sugar for energy. In order to assure that amino acids will build body tissue, carbohydrates must be added to the TPN solution.

Electrolytes and multiple vitamins are added to the TPN solution each day as determined by the individual patient's needs.

Trace elements such as copper, manganese, zinc, and iodide are usually not found in the chemically pure TPN solution. Following prolonged therapy, the patient may show signs of depletion, and, as such, these must be replaced. Zinc deficits have been related to delayed wound healing (Hager, 1977).

INTRALIPID SOLUTION

Fat, in the form of 10% intralipid solution, supplies 9 calories per gram, hence extra calories for more energy. Patients on prolonged TPN therapy may develop fatty-acid deficiencies, and therefore in some patients this therapy is beneficial.

The intralipid solution may be administered as part of the TPN formula. It may be administered intravenously by way of peripheral or central venous lines. Ten percent intralipid is an isotonic solution and therefore suitable for peripheral veins. It may be adminstered concurrently with the TPN solution. Ten percent intralipid solution should neither be filtered nor mixed with other substances.

The dosage of 10% intralipid is 2 g/kg body weight. Initially 1 ml per minute is administered for the first 15 to 30 minutes of therapy. If no untoward reactions occur, the rate can be increased so that 500 ml will be infused over a 4-hour period. Serum lipid profiles should be used in determining subsequent doses.

Caution should be exercised in administering intralipids to patients with severe liver damage, pulmonary disease, anemia, blood coagulation disorders, or when there is a danger of fat embolism.

Some of the adverse reactions of intralipid therapy include dyspnea, cyanosis, urticaria, hyperlipidemia, hypercoagulability, nausea, vomiting, headache, elevated temperature, and back and chest pain. Delayed reactions include hepatomegaly, splenomegaly, thrombocytopenia, leukopenia, transient increases in liver function tests, and overload syndrome (Cutter Laboratories).

PREPARATION OF TPN SOLUTION

The physician uses the patient's disease process, age, weight, and baseline laboratory reports as a guide in determining what ingredients the solution should contain. For the adult the daily amount of solution prescribed is from 2,000 to 4,000 ml.

Following assessment of the patient's needs, the physician writes a prescription or a formula. Some agencies have standard formulas and special formulas, and as such the physician's order will reflect this.

Since the TPN solution is an excellent medium for bacterial growth, it should be prepared under a laminar flow hood (Fig. 7-1). This is best done by a pharmacist who has received special training.

All additives should be filtered of particulate matter, and extreme caution should be taken in order to avoid incompatibilities.

Once prepared and labeled, the solution is refrigerated until 30 to 60 minutes prior to use. It is recommended that solutions be used within 24 hours from the time of preparation. A unit of TPN costs approximately $80, and as such, wastage should be avoided.

Commercially prepared TPN kits are available (Fig. 7-2). These kits contain 500 ml 50% dextrose in a 1000 ml container, 500 ml 8.5% crystalline amino acid solution in a 500 ml container, a solution transfer set, and administration set. Once the dextrose and amino acid solutions are

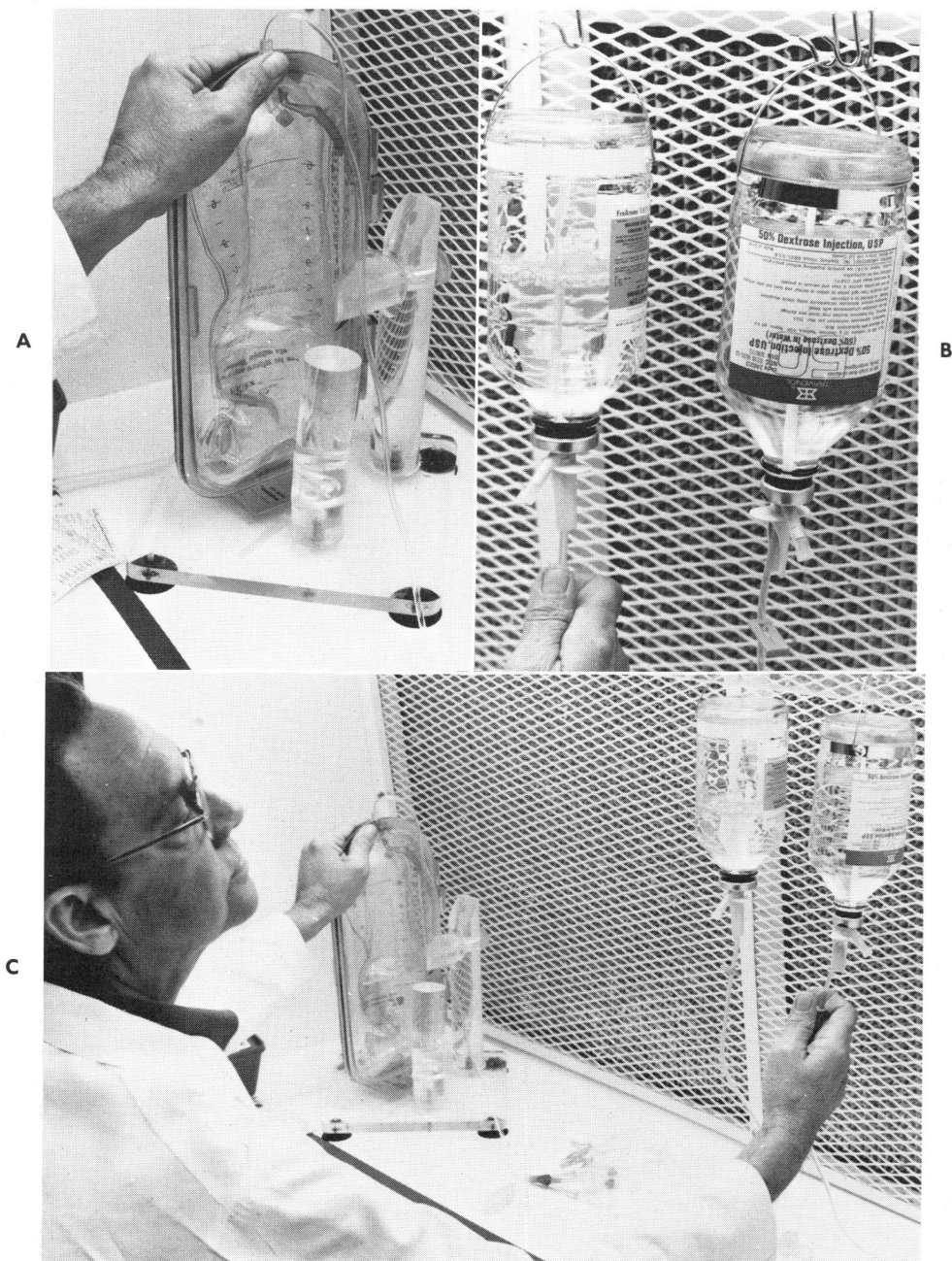

Fig. 7-1. Preparation of TPN solution under laminar flow hood. (Courtesy Alton Ochsner Medical Foundation, New Orleans.)

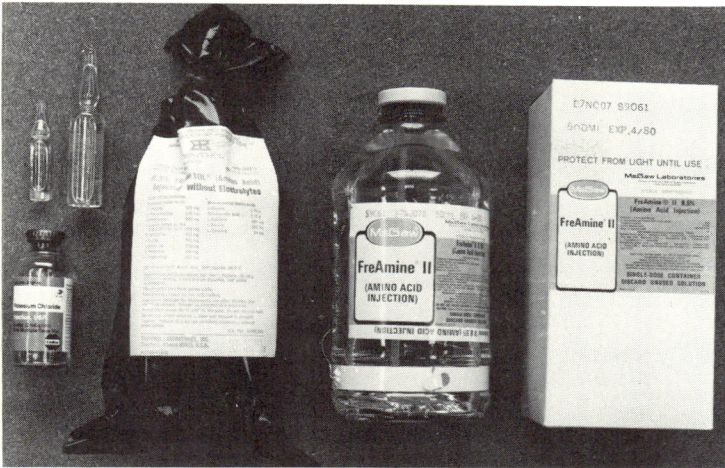

Fig. 7-2. Commercial TPN kit. (Courtesy Alton Ochsner Medical Foundation, New Orleans.)

Name _____	Bag no. _____	
Room no. _____	Rx. no. _____	
FreAmine II (8.5%)		_____ ml
D-50-W		_____ ml
NaCl	_____ mEq	_____ ml
K acetate	_____ mEq	_____ ml
KCl	_____ mEq	_____ ml
Na acetate	_____ mEq	_____ ml
MgSO4 50%	_____ mEq	_____ ml
K phosphate	_____ mm	_____ ml
Ca gluconate	_____ g	_____ ml
Vitamins	_____	_____ ml
Inf. rate _____ ml/hr _____ drops/min		

mixed, other additives such as electrolytes and vitamins are added to the solution.

The boxed material indicates the contents of a typical TPN solution.

The solution and container should be checked for discoloration, clouding, and cracks prior to hanging.

Waterclocking or time-taping of the container and the use of an infusion controller is advisable in order to assure a constant and even flow of the solution.

Should intralipid therapy be ordered to be administered concurrently with the TPN solution, the intralipid solution is connected to the side arm of the TPN solution tubing proximal to the patient. The intralipid solution tubing contains a check valve that prevents the backflow of the intralipid solution into the TPN solution tubing. In addition, the infusion controller, if used, assures that the intralipid solution will flow into the patient. Mixing of the intralipid solution with the TPN solution is minimal and considered safe, since the mixing that occurs is near the tubing and cannula junction.

INSERTION OF SUBCLAVIAN CATHETER FOR ADMINISTERING TPN

Venipuncture of central veins is the responsibility of the physician. The following discussion describes insertion of a subclavian catheter for the purpose of administering TPN. The physician's and nurse's points of view is considered.

Physician's point of view

Subclavian catheter insertion employs a percutaneous puncture of the right or left subclavian vein with cannulation using a polyethylene tubing.

INDICATIONS

Indications include the following: central venous pressure monitoring, administration of TPN, unavailable peripheral veins for cannulation, life-threatening trauma when rapid and massive infusions and transfusions are needed, cardiac arrest, septicemia with gram-negative shock, pulmonary arteriography, insertion of a transvenous pacemaker, and hypovolemia.

EQUIPMENT

Equipment needed for the procedure includes the following (Fig. 7-3): a 14-gauge 8-inch in-the-needle catheter with needle holder, 20 ml syringe, ½- and 2-inch adhesive tape, 4-0 atraumatic silk suture, hemostat, suture scissors and needle holder, shaving kit, 4 × 4 sponges, 3 ml syringe with 25-gauge ⅝-inch needle, gown, gloves, mask cap, anti-infective prepping solution, lidocaine 1% (local anesthetic), antimicrobial ointment, 30-inch extension tubing, 0.22 μm final filter, IV standard, 1000 ml 5% dextrose in water with microdrop tubing, towels,

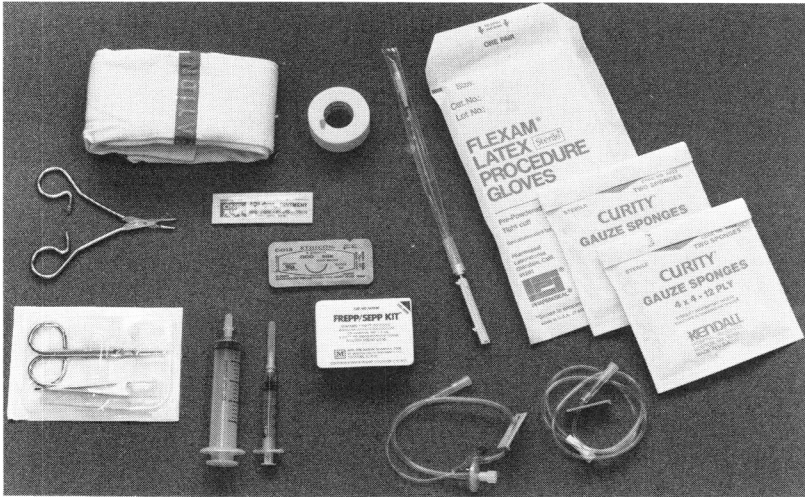

Fig. 7-3. Basic equipment for insertion of subclavian catheter. (Courtesy Alton Ochsner Medical Foundation, New Orleans.)

central venous pressure manometer (optional), infusion controller, and TPN solution. (It is assumed that all equipment is sterile with the exception of mask, cap, IV standard, and infusion controller.)

TECHNIQUE

The methods of approaching the subclavian vein is by supraclavicular or intraclavicular catheterization.

After adequately preparing the particular clavicular area to be used, sterile towels are placed around the prepared site. Local anesthetic is infiltrated into the desired puncture site. The 14-gauge in-the-needle catheter is inserted under the clavicle and advanced into the subclavian vein. Backflow of blood indicates entry. At this point the catheter is threaded into the lumen of the subclavian vein and the wire stylet withdrawn from the catheter. The catheter is then attached to the 5% dextrose solution with previously attached and primed microdrop tubing with extension and filter. The solution is allowed to flow at a fast rate in order to clear the tubing and catheter of blood and then slowed to a keep-open rate.

A solution of 5% or 10% dextrose in water may be used in order to aid the body in adjusting to the forthcoming highly concentrated TPN solution.

The 14-gauge needle is withdrawn and locked into its protective holder. This holder prevents the needle from severing the catheter. The

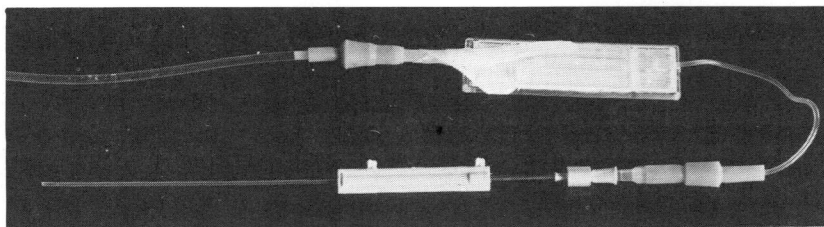

Fig. 7-4. Secured tubing junctions to prevent disconnection and possible air embolism. (Courtesy Alton Ochsner Medical Foundation, New Orleans.)

needle at the catheter junction and at the catheter hub is secured in place with two skin sutures. Antimicrobial ointment is applied at the catheter insertion site and suture sites. A serile occlusive dressing is applied and a chest x-ray is taken to verify catheter placement.

ASSISTANCE REQUIRED FROM NURSE

The nurse is required to assist in shaving and prepping the proposed catheter insertion site, positioning of the patient, preparing the particular intravenous fluids with attached tubing and filter, checking the list of equipment that is necessary prior to the introduction of the catheter, and close observation of the patient following insertion of the catheter for complications.

POSTINSERTION NURSING CARE

Postinsertion nursing care consists of close observation for the development of complications, assuring that tubing junctions are secure and thereby preventing their disconnecting (Fig. 7-4), maintenance of the catheter and catheter site, and administration of the solution as prescribed.

COMPLICATIONS

Complications of subclavian venipuncture include air embolism; subcutaneous emphysema; brachial plexus palsy; septicemia; laceration of the subclavian vein with possible pneumothorax, hydrothorax, or hemothorax; phlebitis and thrombophlebitis; and severed catheter with resulting catheter embolism.

SIGNS AND SYMPTOMS

The signs and symptoms of subclavian catheter complications include dyspnea and severe shortness of breath, chest pain, hematoma overlying the catheter site, spiking temperature with redness and erythema overlying the catheter site, inability to adequately manipulate the arm on the side of the catheter site, edema of the arm, and hypo-tension.

Nurse's point of view

Prior to initiating TPN therapy, it is important for the patient to understand the procedure and why it is being performed. The thought of not eating for several weeks frightens and depresses most patients. The nurse can allay many of these fears with a clear explanation of the proposed therapy.

Before the catheterization procedure begins, instruct the patient in how to perform the Valsalva maneuver. This is done by taking a deep breath and then pushing the air outwardly, as if exhaling, but with the throat and mouth closed. This maneuver increases intrathoracic pressure and aids in preventing air to be inhaled until the subclavian catheter is connected to the infusion tubing, thus preventing air embolism. Ask the patient to practice this a few times before the procedure begins. If the patient is unable to perform the Valsalva maneuver, the nurse is to apply pressure over the patient's abdomen at the appropriate time during the procedure.

The designated area is shaved and prepped as this is considered to be a surgical procedure. Depilatory agents are sometimes used to remove hair from the catheter insertion site.

EQUIPMENT

Preparation of the equipment includes attaching the initial infusion solution to its tubing and filter, priming it, and having all previously listed equipment available and ready for use. It is advisable for the nurse to wear a mask as she or he assists the physician during this procedure. A cap and sterile gown should also be worn, although this is not always feasible.

PROCEDURE

The patient is placed in a supine position with a rolled sheet or towel under the vertebral column to hyperextend the shoulders. The bed should be flat or in a Trendelenburg position to facilitate filling and dilation of the subclavian vein. The patient's head should be turned opposite to the proposed insertion site in order to facilitate access to the site.

Assist the physician with preparation of the skin and injection of the local anesthetic.

After the needle has been inserted and a flow of blood obtained, instruct the patient to perform the Valsalva maneuver. While the patient performs the maneuver, the physician removes the wire stylet from the catheter and, with the assistance of the nurse, connects the catheter to the infusion tubing. The nurse regulates the tubing clamp to deliver the infusion fluid at a fast rate to clear the tubing and catheter of blood. The nurse then regulates the infusion at the prescribed rate.

The catheter is then sutured in place, antimicrobial ointment applied, and an occlusive sterile dressing is placed over the site. The dressing is labeled with the catheter size and length, date, and time of insertion.

The patient is then placed in a comfortable position.

A chest x-ray is obtained to verify the correct positioning of the catheter. Complications of pneumothorax, hydrothorax, or hemothorax may be evident at this time.

Under no circumstances should the TPN solution be started without x-ray verification of correct catheter placement. The nurse should remind the physician should he or she fail to order an x-ray film. In some agencies the x-ray study is part of the procedure, and, as such, a specific order would not be necessary.

Routes of administration for TPN are the right or left subclavian vein. These sites are most commonly used because of mobility, comfort, and longevity. Alternate routes of administration are the right or left internal or external jugular vein, and a catheter threaded from a vein in the antecubital fossa into the superior vena cava.

Since TPN solutions are excellent media for bacterial growth, and since the protein additives are considered to be incompatible with many substances, it is best to avoid using the TPN route for any other purpose such as central venous pressure monitoring and administration of blood and other fluids and medications. A second infusion site should be used for these extra therapies.

Should central venous pressure monitoring become necessary and the TPN route is the available site, it is best to take the readings between TPN solution container changes. This is accomplished by connecting a solution of 0.9% saline solution with the attached central venous pressure manometer following completion of a unit of TPN solution, obtaining the reading, and then connecting the next unit of TPN solution.

GENERAL INFORMATION

The initial rate of flow for TPN solutions is 60 to 80 ml per hour. As the patient's body adapts to the solution, the rate is increased. Rates of flow are determined by the physician.

A baseline weight should be obtained and the patient should be weighed each day in order to ensure that the weight is not shifting rapidly because of fluid gain or loss.

The rate of flow must be constant in order to achieve maximum use of nutrients and metabolic efficiency. If the solution is ordered to run at 80 ml per hour, it should proceed at this rate. Rapid infusion by "catching up" causes marked elevation of serum glucose followed by severe osmotic diuresis and dehydration. If the infusion is behind schedule, the physician should be notified so that schedule alterations can be made. Should the physician approve "catching up," the speed should not exceed 10% of the 24-hour amount ordered. "Catch-up" speeds exceeding this can produce cardiopulmonary overload due to hypervolemia and periods of hyperglycemia alternating with periods of hypoglycemia.

Complications are also caused by sudden slowing down of flow rates, producing hypoglycemia; allergic reactions, especially to protein hydrolysate, which is manifested by fever and other allergic responses; fever from other causes such as infection from a contaminated catheter, tubing, or solution; and insulin shock, unless the patient is slowly tapered off prior to discontinuation of the therapy.

Daily laboratory studies of electrolytes and glucose are generally done. Blood cultures may be ordered at the first sign of septicemia.

Urine tests for sugar and acetone are done every 4 to 6 hours. Testing for sugar should be done with test-tape as opposed to tablets, since TPN solutions cause false-positive readings with tablets.

Emotional depression from prolonged restriction of oral intake, the patient's disease, and extensive hospitalization tend to make the patient feel worthless, rejected, apprehensive, and anxious. The nurse should respond to these psychologic difficulties. Diversive activities are often helpful.

Proper maintenance of the catheter site protects the patient from infection and ensures the catheter's maximum indwelling time. It is advisable to change the site dressing, using strict aseptic technique, every 48 hours. Sometimes the dressing is changed more frequently as indicated by soiling or moisture.

Repeated observation of the site by the same pair of eyes can assure recognition of changes in appearance that may indicate infection. It is recommended that the same nurse change the dressing each time. The first signs of inflammation, purulence, thrombophlebitis, or extravasation warrant removal of the catheter.

Cleaning the site includes removal of the dressing, donning of sterile gloves and face mask, defatting the skin with 70% isopropyl alcohol, inspection of the site for leakage, redness, edema, and general condition, application of a suitable antimicrobial ointment, and application of a new sterile dressing. The dressing is labeled with the catheter size and length, date changed, and nurse's name.

The infusion tubing and 0.22 μm final filter should be changed every 8 to 12 hours or with each additional unit of TPN solution. All tubing junctions should be taped securely in order to protect them from accidentally disconnecting. All air is removed from the tubing and filter, and the Valsalva maneuver is performed while the tubing is being changed.

Temperatures should be checked and recorded every 4 hours. Any unexplained fever should be investigated. The physician should examine the patient and initiate appropriate diagnostic measures to determine the cause of the fever. A temperature spike of 39.4 C (103 F) with chills may be indicative of a febrile reaction. Solution and catheter cultures are sometimes necessary in determining the cause of fever.

Catheter occlusion should be reported to the physician. He or she may elect to irrigate the catheter with normal saline in an effort to clear the catheter. Strict aseptic technique should be adhered to.

Should the patient complain of shoulder or neck pain, or should the nurse note supraclavicular edema, the physician should be notified. This may indicate extravasation of fluid, thrombophlebitis, or thrombus formation.

Signs and symptoms of hyperglycemia include nausea, headache, lassitude, glycosuria, and diuresis. Signs and symptoms of hypoglycemia include confusion, restlessness, diaphoresis, general muscular weakness, tremors, twitching, and epigastric cramping. These signs and symptoms should be observed and the physician notified should they occur. Nonketotic diabetic coma may occur.

Scurvy, rickets, and other conditions related to vitamin deficiencies may occur. Signs and symptoms of these should be reported to the physician.

Observe for and report signs and symptoms of dehydration, overhydration, or circulatory overload. These include dryness of mucous membranes, decreased urinary output, dry skin, productive cough with frothy sputum, full bounding pulse, increased urinary output, and overdistended neck veins.

References

Beland, I., and Passos, J.: Clinical nursing, ed. 3, New York, 1975, Macmillan Publishing Co.

Cutter Laboratories: 10% intralipid, product information, Berkeley, Calif., 1976, Cutter Laboratories.

Hager, E.: Drug intelligence and clinical pharmacology, vol. 11, Hamilton, Ill., March 1977, Hamilton Press.

Kaminski, M.: Hyperalimentation: who, what, and why, Surg. Team Mag. **5:**3, June 1976.

Smith, Kline, and French Laboratories: Total parenteral nutrition, New York, 1975, Smith, Kline, and French Laboratories.

Chapter 8

Blood therapy

From the beginning of time blood has been thought of as a mystical power. Egyptians once bathed in blood as it was considered to purify and cure (Flexner, 1967). It was only after the discovery of circulation by Harvey in the early seventeenth century that blood as a living and circulating tissue became a topic of scientific study (Abbott, 1966).

Blood was first successfully transfused from one living person to another during World War I, while the first recorded yet unsuccessful person-to-person transfusion occurred in the year 1492.

Prior failures can be attributed to the transfusion of nonhuman blood such as that of sheep and oxen, use of contaminated and coagulated blood, lack of appropriate equipment, inadequate storage facilities and techniques, and the use of incompatible blood, since the Rhesus (Rh) factor, blood typing, and cross-matching had not yet been discovered.

The concept of successful transfusions became a reality in 1901 when Landsteiner discovered the ABO system, a method of classifying antigens and isoagglutinins (antibodies) in the red blood cells and serum (Plumer, 1975). Houston is credited with discovering the anticoagulant sodium citrate in 1914.

Blood banking commenced in 1937 when Cook County General Hospital of Chicago set up the first blood bank.

During the years between World Wars I and II, fractionation of blood became popular when it was realized that the benefits achieved from receiving components of blood far outweighed those achieved from simple whole blood replacement, regardless of what the deficiency was. This paved the way for physicians to treat a specific disease entity with a specific component, fraction, or part of whole blood.

In the United States over six million patients receive some form of blood therapy each year. It is estimated that 3,000 patients die each year as a result of blood therapy complications. This is approximately

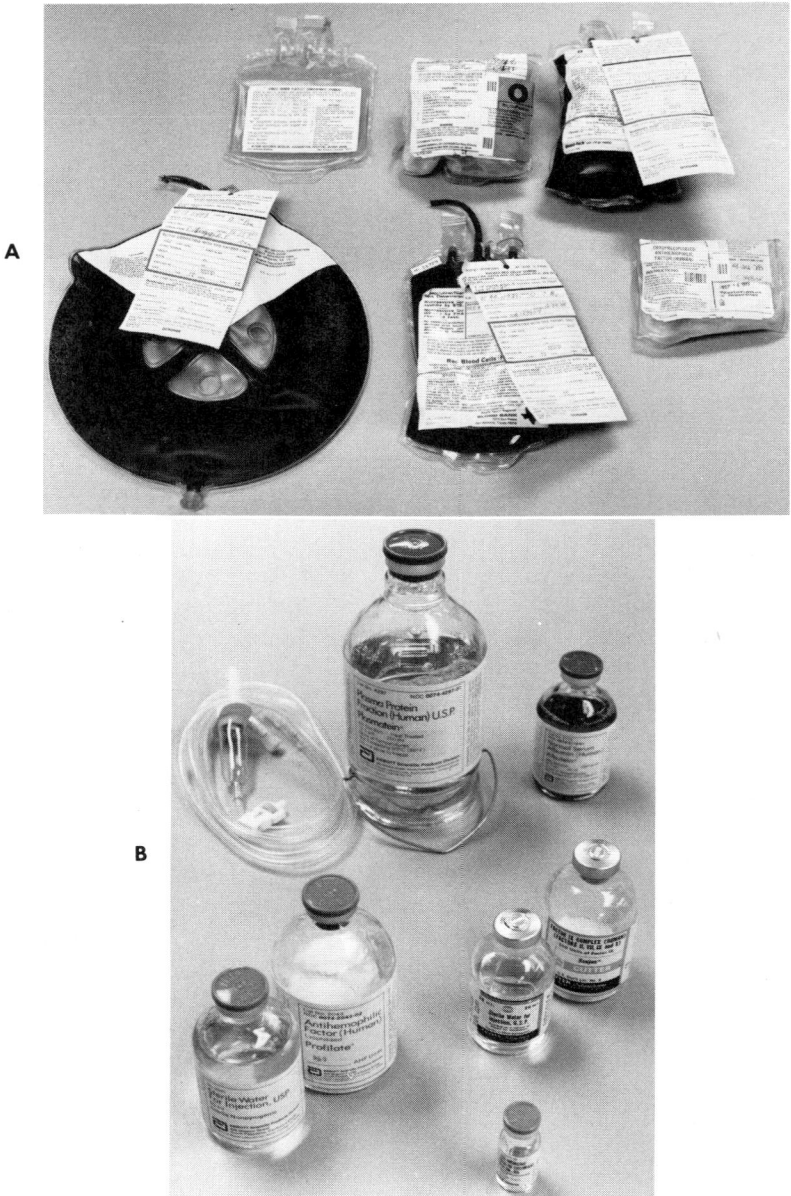

Fig. 8-1. A, Blood. **B,** Blood components. (Courtesy Alton Ochsner Medical Foundation, New Orleans.)

1 in 5,000 and about the same number who die from the untoward effects of general anesthesia.

One unit of whole blood raises the average adult's hemoglobin level by 1 to 1½ g/100 ml and the hematocrit by 2% to 3%.

Whole blood is made up of two basic components: cellular or particulate matter and plasma (Flexner, 1967) (Fig. 8-1). The cellular component comprises approximately 45% of the blood. It is composed primarily of erythrocytes, leukocytes, and platelets. The plasma comprises approximately 55% of the blood. It is about 90% water (serum) and 7% protein (albumin, globulin, and fibrogen). About 1% to 3% of the plasma is made up of such things as lipids, electrolytes, vitamins, carbohydrates, nonprotein nitrogenous compounds, bilirubin, and gases.

Plasma is the liquid part of blood. In the blood, erythrocytes, leukocytes, and platelets float in plasma. Plasma is the medium for circulation of blood cells. It carries nutritive substances to various structures and removes waste products of metabolism from those structures (Thomas, 1977).

Normal plasma is thin and colorless when free from corpuscles, or it has a faint yellow tinge. After clotting of blood, the liquid squeezed out by the clot is called blood serum. Serum is the watery portion of blood.

If whole blood is prevented from clotting either by chilling or by adding anticoagulants, it can be centrifuged. The clear fluid that then occupies the upper half of the centrifuge tube is called plasma.

The trend in blood therapy is the administration of fractionated blood components as opposed to whole blood per se because the danger of overloading the patient's circulatory system can most often be prevented. Careful consideration is given to the patient's specific deficit and that deficit is replaced. Studies and logic show that the benefits from component replacement are far superior to the former method of administering whole blood for all deficits. In addition, rising hospital costs can to a degree be controlled, since one unit of whole blood can be fractionated and serve several patients.

Whole blood can be fractionated into red blood cells, platelet suspensions and concentrates, leukocytes, fresh plasma, frozen and stored plasma, albumin, cryoprecipitates or factor VIII concentrates, fibrinogen, gamma globulin, and factors II, VII, IX, and X concentrates.

Blood banks in today's hospitals are far more sophisticated than ever before. Blood bank directors are board-certified pathologists. Blood bank technologists are medical technologists with 1 to 2 years postgraduate study in immunohematology and blood banking.

Nurses should consider blood bankers as indispensable members of the health care team. Without their expertise, support, and guidance, quality care would be difficult to deliver.

The United States government passed a law that prevents blood from being sold to blood banks by donors. This law has made it difficult for blood banks to obtain adequate supplies of blood. With effective donor recruitment programs within agencies and freezing of blood, shortages have been to a degree curtailed.

One unit of whole blood costs approximately $40, and a regular blood container with its added anticoagulant acid buffer and sugar costs approximately $6. Price ranges for whole blood and its components vary within the United States.

The basic purposes of blood or blood component therapy are to maintain blood volume and its coagulation properties by supplying red blood cells and clotting factors.

The specific reasons for administering blood and its components, approximate volume of each unit, shelf life, and general information regarding each follows.

WHOLE BLOOD

Whole blood is administered to maintain or replace lost volume during hemorrhagic emergencies and, when fresh, can supply needed coagulation properties during these periods. The approximate volume of one unit of whole blood is 500 ml. Each unit contains CPD (sodium citrate as coagulant, citric acid as buffer, and dextrose to assist with metabolic processes and prolong the life of the cells) (Plumer, 1975).

If properly refrigerated at 1 to 6 C (33.8 to 42.8 F), the shelf life of whole blood is 21 days. With age, potassium escapes from the red blood cells into the plasma, thus increasing plasma potassium to 23 mEq/liter by the twenty-first day. This high potassium content of the plasma can produce cardiac arrest should massive transfusions be needed. Platelets and other coagulation factors are altered, and waste products of cell metabolism such as microaggregates of leukocytes, platelets, and other materials develop, predisposing the recipient to pulmonary insufficiency (Plumer, 1975). This is one reason for considering using microaggregate filters rather than the traditional filters during blood administration.

Citrate additives can cause calcium deficits.

RED BLOOD CELLS

Red blood cells or packed red blood cells are administered to correct acute and chronic anemias not responsive to specific therapy, preoperative anemia not correctable with medications or time available, and bone marrow failure due to malignancies. Red blood cells are also administered to patients with renal, hepatic, or circulatory impairment, patients who are elderly or debilitated to prevent overload, and burned patients with hyperkalemia.

Since plasma is removed from red blood cells, there is a smaller amount of electrolytes, agglutinins, ammonium, and citrate than in whole blood. The reduced sodium is beneficial to cardiac patients and the reduced potassium is beneficial to renal patients. Another reason for using red blood cells is to maintain the oxygen carrying capacity of the blood by supplying erythrocytes without the danger of overloading the patient.

Red blood cells are prepared by removing 200 to 225 ml of plasma from one unit of whole blood. The shelf life is 21 days.

LEUKOCYTE-POOR BLOOD

Leukocyte-poor blood is administered to renal patients who are candidates for transplants, since it prevents sensitization to tissue antigens, and to patients who have developed leukoagglutinins, since it helps in preventing febrile reactions.

The shelf life is 21 days or 24 hours after the unit is opened. The volume of one unit is 200 to 250 ml.

Leukocyte-poor blood is produced by removing leukocytes and platelets from whole blood. This must be done while the blood is fresh. The process includes saline washing and sedimentation or centrifugation. Electrolytes are lost. It can be obtained from frozen red blood cells, since most leukocytes and platelets are removed during the freezing process. The risk of hepatitis is the same as with whole blood.

FROZEN BLOOD CELLS

Frozen blood cells are administered, after thawing, as autologous transfusions for patients whose surgery is scheduled at least 1 month in advance, to patients who are scheduled for organ transplants, to patients who have repeated febrile reactions, and to provide blood for those patients with antibodies to high-incidence antigens where it may be difficult to obtain compatible blood.

Frozen red blood cells provide a stockpile of blood of selected types for use when banked blood may be in short supply.

The shelf life is 3 years frozen and 24 hours thawed. The volume of one unit is 200 ml.

A glycerol solution is added to the red blood cells prior to freezing. Glycerol acts as a cryoprotective agent. Freezing arrests cell metabolism. Prior to administration the cells are thawed and the glycerol is washed out. The benefits to the patient are the same as fresh red blood cells; however, the process is expensive. Washing removes blood leukocytes, platelets, group antibodies, microaggregates, plasma proteins, electrolytes, toxic products, and some if not all of the hepatitis virus. The risk of hepatitis is less than with whole blood.

PLATELETS

Platelets are administered for the purpose of treating bleeding thrombocytopenia, the effectiveness of which is diminished during acute hemorrhage; transfusion reactions; marked splenomegaly; idiopathic thrombocytopenia purpura; when platelet agglutinins are formed after multiple platelet transfusions; treatment of patients with chronic depletion of platelets due to certain diseases such as leukemia, aplastic anemia, and other forms of cancer; and patients with mild thrombocytopenia who are to undergo major surgical procedures.

Platelets are extracted from whole blood manually or by plateletpheresis (Rossman and associates, 1977). Plateletpheresis is described as the separation and removal of platelets from whole blood by centrifugation and returning the remainder to the donor.

The shelf life for platelets is 6 to 72 hours. The actual shelf life depends on storage techniques. The volume of each unit is 10 to 50 ml. Ten milliliters of platelets will raise the recipient's platelet count by 5000 cu mm. A level of 30,000 is usually adequate in preventing severe hemorrhage; therefore six to eight units is considered an adequate dose (Brunner and Suddarth, 1975).

Platelets should be administered as rapidly as possible. Prophylactic administration may cause alloimmunization, which may limit effectiveness of later therapy.

The risk of hepatitis is the same as with whole blood.

PLASMA

Plasma is administered for the purpose of treating clotting factor deficiencies when specific concentrates are not available or when the precise factor deficiency has not been determined.

Plasma is separated from whole blood within 4 hours of collection. It contains all of the plasma clotting factors. Freezing preserves the clotting factors and, unless administered immediately after thawing, factor VIII (the antihemophiliac factor, AHF) will be lost (Plumer, 1975).

Plasma is dispensed as liquid, frozen, and dried (lyophilized). Single-donor fresh-frozen plasma and single-donor fresh plasma contain all of the clotting factors; however, factors V and VIII will be lost on storage in the nonfrozen state. These must be compatible with the recipient's ABO group.

The shelf life in single-donor liquid plasma is 3 years, frozen plasma 1 to 5 years, and freeze-dried (lyophilized) plasma 7 years.

The risk of hepatitis with plasma is the same as with whole blood.

SINGLE-DONOR FACTOR VIII-RICH CRYOPRECIPITATE AND ANTIHEMOPHILIA CONCENTRATE (AHF, AHG)

Single-donor factor VIII–rich cryoprecipitate and antihemophilia concentrate (AHF, AHG) is administered for the purpose of treating hemophilia, von Willebrand's disease, fibrinogen deficiency, and factor XIII deficiency (American Association of Blood Banks, 1975).

It is prepared by extracting the precipitated factor VIII from a thawed unit of fresh-frozen plasma. The volume of each container is 10 to 25 ml. Contained in each 10 to 25 ml are 80 to 100 units of factor VIII, the von Willebrand's factor, factor XIII (fibrin stabilizing factor, FSF), small amounts of fibrinogen, factor II (prothrombin), factor V (proaccelerin), factor V (proconvertin), factor IX (PTC), factor X (Stuart-Prower), and factor XII (Hageman).

A unit is defined as that amount of activity present in 1 ml of normal fresh plasma (American Association of Blood Banks, 1975).

The shelf life is 1 year frozen and 4 to 6 hours thawed. The risk of hepatitis is the same as with whole blood.

FACTOR II THROUGH X COMPLEX

Factor II through X complex contains factors II, VII, IX, and X. It is administered for the purpose of correcting deficiencies of the factors it contains and to prevent hemorrhage during surgery. It is especially useful for patients with hemophilia B or Christmas disease (factor IX deficiency). It is a lyophilized preparation. The shelf life is 6 months. The risk of hepatitis is so great that its use should be restricted.

FIBRINOGEN

Fibrinogen is administered for the purpose of treating fibrinogen deficiencies. It is derived from pooled plasma. The shelf life is 5 years. The risk of hepatitis is greater than with whole blood. It is sometimes preferred to use cryoprecipitate in its place (American Association of Blood Banks, 1975). Consideration is being given to discontinuing the manufacture of fibrinogen.*

---

*FDA discontinued fibrinogen in 1978. (Food and Drug Administration Drug Bulletin, Oct.-Nov., 1978.)

ALBUMIN AND PLASMA PROTEIN FRACTION

Albumin and plasma protein fraction is available in a 5% buffered saline solution and a 25% "salt-poor" form. As of February 1978 the Food and Drug Administration required that all 25% normal serum albumin (human) must have a range of sodium content between 130 and 160 mEq/liter. A Food and Drug Administration bulletin of November 1978 required that the labeling of 25% normal serum albumin (human) must no longer include the terms "salt-poor," since this term is a misnomer that has persisted since high-salt products containing 300 mEq of sodium chloride per liter disappeared from the market over 30 years ago (Food and Drug Administration Drug Bulletin, Oct.-Nov., 1978).

This substance is administered for the purpose of treating hemorrhagic shock, trauma, and infection when plasma volume expansion is desired.

It is desirable to use the 25% solution to treat hypoproteinemia and cerebral edema.

The volume of each unit is 50 to 250 ml. The shelf life is 3 to 5 years. The risk of hepatitis is less than with whole blood.

These preparations should not be administered through total parenteral nutrition lines containing protein hydrolysate or alcohol, since a precipitate may form.

Circulatory overload and pulmonary edema are side effects.

IMMUNE SERUM GLOBULIN AND SPECIFIC IMMUNOGLOBULINS

Immune serum globulin and specific immunoglobulins, although administered intramuscularly, are included here.

These substances are administered for the purpose of providing temporary immunity to conditions such as agammaglobulinemia, hypogammaglobulinemia, tetanus, pertussis, mumps, measles, herpes, chickenpox, and smallpox exposure. The shelf life is from 1 to 3 years. The risk of hepatitis is less than with whole blood (Beland and Passos, 1975).

Included in this series is $Rh_0(D)$ globulin. It is administered for the purpose of preventing anti-$Rh_0(D)$ antibodies in the Rh_0-negative individual who has received Rh_0-positive blood following delivery or abortion of an $Rh_0(D)$-positive infant or fetus, or following receiving a transfusion of $Rh_0(D)$-positive blood.

PLASMA SUBSTITUTES

Plasma substitutes are administered for the purpose of expanding blood volume. Dextran, as an example, is a solution with a molecular weight higher than that of blood. When introduced into the vascular system, osmotic pressure increases, causing osmotic diuresis and a resulting increase in blood volume.

Dextran is sometimes used following total joint replacement surgery. Its ability to alter the electrical charge of blood cells aids in the prevention of blood clots.

Each container contains 500 ml. Filtering is not required. The risk of hepatitis is nil.

The administration of excessive amounts of dextran (greater than 1500 ml) can increase bleeding tendencies. Allergic reactions have been known to occur. It is available in dextrose and saline solutions.

Ringer's lactate solution is administered for the purpose of treating fluid and electrolyte imbalance and metabolic acidosis. The solution contains calories, water, bicarbonate, and lactate. Lactate solutions should not be used in patients with hepatic dysfunction or anoxia due to shock or congestive heart failure (American Association of Blood Banks, 1975).

ADMINISTRATION OF BLOOD
Laws

Many state laws require that only approved registered nurses be allowed to perform all aspects of blood therapy. Approved means that the nurse receives and successfully completes in-service training in blood therapy.

Blood therapy includes ordering blood, checking blood, hanging blood, observing the patient for expected action and reactions, regulating blood, discontinuing blood, obtaining blood samples for type and cross matching, and documenting the therapy as performed.

In some agencies the licensed practical (vocational) nurse is permitted to regulate the flow of blood, observe the patient for expected actions and reactions, discontinue the blood, and document the therapy performed.

It is advisable to be knowledgeable regarding individual state laws and agency policies and to stay within the limits that have been set.

Filters

Blood and its components must be filtered prior to being administered to the patient. This is accomplished while the blood is being administered.

There are two types of filters available. The regular "Y"-type or straight-type blood administration set and the microaggregate filter. The micrometer size of blood filters ranges from 40 to 170 μm.

The microaggregate filter, measured in micrometers, is especially useful when three or more units of blood are being administered and when the blood being administered is not fresh.

The filtering effect of the microaggregate filter is far superior to the regular blood filter. The amount of blood to be administered and the cost to the patient are considerations in selecting blood filters.

It is advisable to change the regular blood administration set with each subsequent unit of blood. At no time should an infusion be connected to a used blood filter, since filtered particles are eventually diluted, dissolved, and dislodged from the filter, causing the filtered particles to be administered to the patient.

Normal saline can be used to clear the tubing of blood following a transfusion. Following clearing, the tubing should be changed and the filter removed.

Prior to using any filter, it should be wetted and flushed with 30 to 60 ml of sterile normal saline. This is done by connecting an infusion container of saline to the tubing and filter. The drip chamber of the regular blood administration set is to be filled ⅔ to ¾ full in order to assure complete wetting of the filter and to reduce the distance in which each drop of blood will fall into the chamber. This will minimize damage to the blood cells. The microaggregate filter is connected between the normal saline container and the regular blood administration set. Both microaggregate and regular blood filters are then wetted.

Once wetting and clearing of the tubing and filter is accomplished the blood is attached. The transfusion may then be started.

Specific directions for connecting and wetting each type of filter can be found on package inserts.

Should blood be followed by an infusion, the tubing is changed, the filter removed, and the needle or cannula is flushed with 10 to 20 ml of normal saline. Flushing of the needle or cannula may be done by attaching a syringe with normal saline to the needle or cannula.

Most blood bankers suggest the use of only normal saline for all flushing and priming procedures related to blood therapy. In some instances Ringer's solution or Ringer's lactate solutions are used. There is a danger of incompatibilities with these solutions, however, and the calcium present in Ringer's solutions may cause clotting.

Permission

Most agencies require a signed, witnessed consent from the patient prior to blood administration. This consent protects the agency, physician, and nurse from litigation. Agency policy regarding preparation, signing, and witnessing of consents should be adhered to.

Typing and cross matching

A physician's order is usually required to obtain a blood sample for typing and cross-matching. In some institutions only the physician, IV nurse, and nurses in intensive and emergency care areas are permitted to obtain blood samples for typing and cross-matching. The rationale is that fewer numbers of persons performing a procedure will result in fewer errors. If for some reason the blood sample is mislabeled, it is possible that the patient may receive the wrong blood. This may cause death.

Checking the blood

Most agencies require that a physician and physician, a physician and registered nurse, or a registered nurse and a registered nurse check blood before it is administered. The blood should be checked by two qualified persons. Any discrepancy regarding information on the blood bag or blood tag should be corrected only by the blood bank staff. This necessitates returning the blood to the bank and delaying the transfusion.

Warming of blood

Warming of blood is usually done when multiple transfusions are required. Portable and stationary blood warmers are available (Fig. 8-2).

Instructions for using blood warmers must be strictly adhered to in order to prevent overwarming and destruction of blood cells.

When mechanical blood warmers are not available, the unit of blood is sometimes placed in a warm water bath. This method of warming is not recommended, since the dangers of overwarming and contamination by seepage of water into the unit of blood are great.

Refrigeration of blood

In order to preserve blood and prevent contamination, blood should be refrigerated at 4 C (39.2 F). Blood refrigerators are continuously monitored so that the appropriate temperature is maintained (Fig. 8-3).

If hanging of blood is delayed beyond 30 minutes from the time it is received from the blood bank, it should be returned to the bank for refrigeration. Ordinary refrigerators are not equipped with the special temperature monitoring devices found on blood refrigerators. As such, the temperature of the nurses' station refrigerator may be too cool or too warm, thereby predisposing the blood cells to freezing or early contamination because of hastened bacterial growth. In either case the possibility of a transfusion reaction increases.

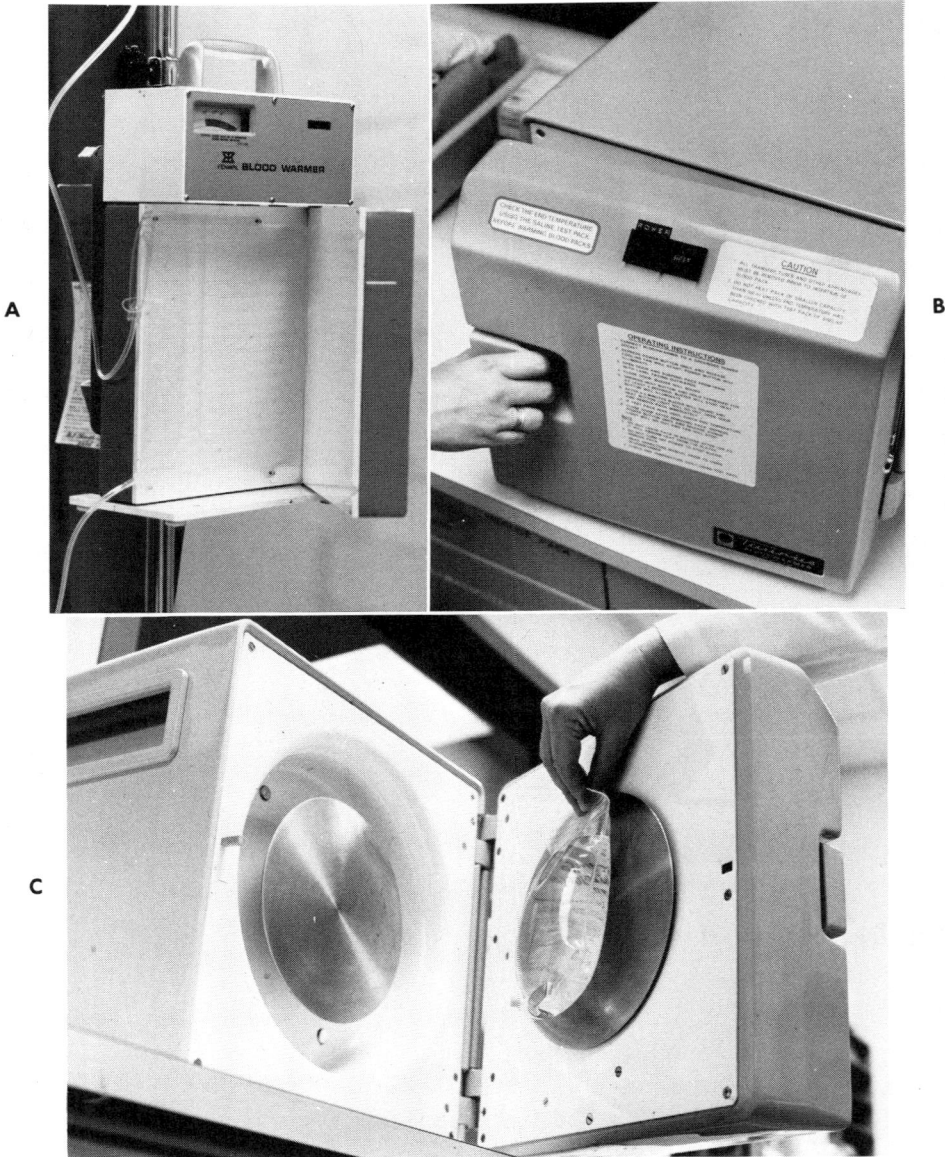

Fig. 8-2. A, Portable blood warmer with plastic tubing and coil attached. **B** and **C,** Outside and inside views of stationary blood warmer. (Courtesy Alton Ochsner Medical Foundation, New Orleans.)

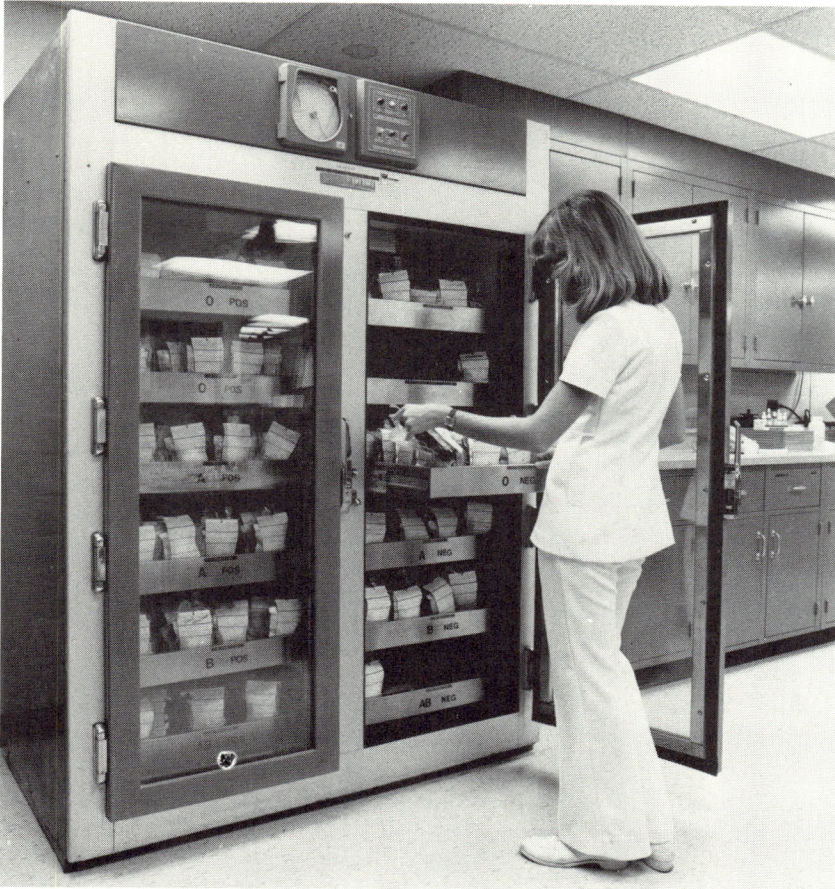

Fig. 8-3. Blood refrigerator. Note special monitoring device above refrigerator doors. (Courtesy Alton Ochsner Medical Foundation, New Orleans.)

Certain special care areas such as operating room suites and intensive care areas may be equipped with blood refrigerators. In such cases, returning the blood to the bank would not be necessary.

Blood bags and tags

The blood tag is to remain on the blood bag until the transfusion is completed. Both bag and tag are to be returned to the blood bank. The used tubing should accompany the bag and tag. This used equipment is stored in the bank for a period of time, since delayed blood reactions do occur and in such cases a sample of blood would be available for analysis.

Intravenous standard

A portable intravenous standard is preferred to those that attach to beds, since greater height of the transfusing blood can be achieved. Because of its viscosity, blood flows best when the distance between the bag and patient exceeds 0.9 m (3 ft).

Blood bag rotation

Since blood is a suspension, it separates on standing. Mixing of this suspension is required prior to administration. This can be accomplished by gently rotating the blood bag several times. Vigorous shaking of the blood bag is not recommended, since this may damage or destroy blood cells.

Patient identification

Transfusing the wrong blood to the wrong patient can lead to death; therefore proper identification is vital.

Identify by checking the blood bag and tag data with the patient's chart and agency (hospital) number, type and cross-match record, identification arm band, and by having the patient state his full name. Ascertain that all information correlates. The blood bag and tag identifying information includes the blood type and Rh factor, donor name, date collected, expiration date, patient (recipient) name, agency (hospital), and room number.

When checking the blood bag and tag, one checker should read the information from the bag while the other checker verifies the information on the tag.

Needle or cannula size

A 19- or 21-gauge needle or cannula is acceptable for peripheral intravenous transfusions. Avoid, whenever possible, needles with gauges smaller than 21, since the viscosity of blood will impede flow rates.

Rates of administration

Avoid contamination of blood by adhering to strict aseptic practices and by transfusing whole blood within 2 to 4 hours, red blood cells within 1 hour, and platelets as rapidly as possible.

Bacterial overgrowth begins 30 minutes following removal from the refrigerator.

Should the blood fail to flow or flow sluggishly, the transfusion should be restarted in another site in order that the blood be administered within the safe time period.

Pumping of blood

When pumping of blood is necessary, a physician's order is required.

Pumping predisposes the patient to air embolism if a vented blood container is used.

Cuff pumping may injure blood cells because of the squeezing action placed on the blood bag. When cuff pumps are used, it is important to keep the pump pressure within the safe range. The safe range is indicated on the pump dial.

Blood reactions

Following the initiation of a transfusion, the blood should be maintained at a keep-open rate for the first 15 to 20 minutes or until the first 50 to 100 ml is administered. Following this, the flow is adjusted to the prescribed rate. It is during this period that most reactions occur. Signs and symptoms of a blood reaction may become evident following the transfusion of as little as 10 ml of blood.

Should untoward effects occur (nausea, vomiting, bone pain, flank pain, palpitations, undue anxiety and apprehension, elevated pulse, urticaria, itching, burning of the face and at the needle site, changes in the blood pressure, weakness, shortness of breath, chills, and fever), discontinue the blood and notify the physician and blood bank immediately.

The vein should be kept open with normal saline while awaiting reaction protocol instructions. The blood and transfusion tubing is to be protected from contamination during this period.

The physician is responsible for determining whether the reaction is true and for what action should be taken.

Platelet administration

Some authorities suggest changing tubings and filters between each unit of platelets, since incompatibilities can occur. In addition, should the patient have a reaction, it would be difficult to determine which unit of platelets caused the reaction.

Should a unit of whole blood or red blood cells be administered between two units of platelets, a separate filter should be used and the needle or cannula should be flushed with normal saline. It is because of the danger of incompatibilities that this is recommended.

Commercially prepared products

Since procedures for administration of commercially prepared products vary, it is advisable to follow the directions on the package insert regarding methods of administration, rates of flow, and filtering.

BLOOD TRANSFUSION PROCEDURE
Equipment

Equipment for blood transfusion includes whole blood or components, blood administration set (regular filter or microaggregate filter), infusion equipment as required, and a portable infusion standard.

Method

1. Check transfusion card against physician's order and initial.
2. Check signing of permit.
3. Check blood label on bag with tag, type and match record for name, agency (hospital) number, bag number, type, donor name, and donation and expiration dates.
4. Sign tag.
5. Compare patient's name and agency (hospital) number on identification armband with blood bag and tag information.
6. Gently rotate bag to distribute blood cells.
7. Prime tubing drip chamber and filter(s) with normal saline.
8. Start infusion.
9. Disconnect normal saline container from tubing.
10. Connect blood to tubing.
11. Run at keep-open rate for first 15 to 20 minutes, then regulate at prescribed rate.
12. Check frequently, every 30 to 60 minutes for rate of flow, infiltration, and side effects.
13. Discontinue when transfusion is completed unless infusion is to be resumed.
14. Return blood bag, tag, and tubing to blood bank.
15. Addition of blood to existing infusion containing solution other than plain normal saline:
    a. Disconnect existing tubing at needle or cannula site.
    b. Flush needle or cannula with syringe containing 10 to 20 ml normal saline.
    c. Connect blood with primed tubing and filter(s) to needle or cannula.
    d. Discontinue when completed.
    e. If infusion is to be resumed, flush needle or cannula with syringe containing 10 to 20 ml normal saline prior to reconnecting infusion.

BLOOD REACTIONS

The nurse administering blood should possess adequate knowledge of the potential dangers involved in blood therapy before she or he attempts to add this therapy to her or his practice.

Included in the nurses' knowledge base regarding blood and its components are indications, usual amounts administered, contraindications, precautions, side effects, toxicity, and antidotes.

Approximately 5% of blood reactions are due to serologic incompatibilities. The majority of these incompatibilities are due to clerical error, that is to say, wrong blood to wrong patient.

Signs and symptoms of mild to moderate reactions include hives, chills, fever, palpitations, chest pain, back pain, flank pain, shortness of breath, headache, flushing, and loss of consciousness.

Signs and symptoms of severe reactions include shock, oliguria, hematuria, borborygmus (a gurgling, splashing sound heard over the large intestine), and a predisposition to several diseases.

Any reaction, no matter how slight, should be considered potentially dangerous and should be treated as an acute medical emergency.

Classification
HEMOLYTIC TRANSFUSION REACTIONS

Hemolytic transfusion reactions occur because of an incompatibility between the transfusing blood and the patient's blood. It is almost always due to human error, and the reaction may begin following the administration of as little as 10 ml of blood.

Signs and symptoms in the initial phase include anxiety, flushing, pleuritic-type chest pain, shortness of breath, tachycardia, and low back pain or pains in the long bones, especially of the femur.

As the reaction progresses the patient becomes febrile. Nausea, vomiting, cyanosis, oliguria, anuria, uremia with shock, blood hemolysis, and death may occur.

HOMOLOGOUS SERUM HEPATITIS (SERUM HEPATITIS OR TYPE B HEPATITIS)

Homologous serum hepatitis occurs when the virus is transmitted by the transfusion of blood and many of its components. The use of contaminated needles, cannulae, tubing, and other equipment during blood therapy may cause hepatitis.

The Australian antigen is a reactant related to type B hepatitis, and its presence in donor blood usually indicates that hepatitis could be transmitted. The incubation period for the type B hepatitis virus is 6 weeks to 6 months. Mortality is from 0.1% to 10%.

Signs and symptoms of this reaction include anorexia, jaundice, dyspepsia, abdominal pain, generalized malaise, and weakness. Hepatomegaly and splenomegaly are common.

Treatment includes bed rest and an adequate diet of vitamin B complex, proteins, and carbohydrates. Recovery may take 4 or more months.

Prevention includes the administration of immune serum globulin. The use of disposable equipment has been beneficial in controlling this reaction.

PYROGENIC REACTIONS

Pyrogenic reactions are caused by bacterial contamination of the blood. The usual organisms involved are gram-negative coliform bacilli, diphtheroid organisms, and staphylococci.

Bacteremic shock develops and death follows the administration of as little as 25 ml of contaminated blood. Improved refrigeration and the use of disposable equipment has curbed pyrogenic reactions to a great extent.

A unit of blood can be considered suspect should the container appear overfilled. This is caused by a collection of gas due to bacterial overgrowth.

ALLERGIC REACTIONS

Allergic reactions occur as the recipient responds to the donor blood. The donor may have ingested substances such as medications or foods that the recipient is allergic to.

Signs and symptoms include itching, hives, and asthma. Allergic reactions are usually treated with antihistamines.

CIRCULATORY OVERLOAD

Rather than a blood reaction, circulatory overload is considered to be a response due to hypervolemia.

OVERTRANSFUSION REACTION

Overtransfusion reactions usually occur when patients receive massive transfusion therapy. Eight to ten or more units of blood administered to a patient are considered massive therapy. Hemorrhage becomes uncontrollable, since a platelet washout occurs. This can be controlled by administering fresh whole blood or platelets in conjunction with whole blood therapy.

CITRATE INTOXICATION

Citrate intoxication usually occurs when patients receive massive transfusion therapy. Intoxication occurs especially when the liver is unable to metabolize the citrate. It produces convulsions, impaired clotting, hyperpotassemia with cardiac irritability and arrest, and ammonia intoxication with stupor and coma.

RAPID PRESSURE REACTION

Rapid pressure reactions occur during massive transfusions of cold blood. It produces general hypothermia and cardiac arrest. This reaction can be prevented by administering warmed blood.

ZUCKER'S PLATELET WASHOUT PHENOMENON

Zucker's platelet washout phenomenon is a hemorrhagic catastrophe occurring when large amounts of nonfresh blood are administered. This blood is relatively free of platelets and therefore, unless platelet supplements are provided for in the form of extracted platelets or by using fresh whole blood, the patient will "bleed out."

FEBRILE AND URTICARIAL REACTIONS

Febrile and urticarial reactions occur in some patients and are not considered life-threatening. The treatment protocol is symptomatic.

DELAYED REACTIONS

Delayed reactions occur several days to 2 weeks following the administration of blood. The treatment depends on the reaction.

Blood reaction protocol

Caution and preventive measures are vital in transfusions. Nonetheless, a reaction can occur, even a severe one. In the event of a reaction, several steps are essential.

Reaction protocol includes discontinuing the blood and keeping the vein open with normal saline, notifying the physician and the blood bank, monitoring vital signs and urinary output, treating shock, obtaining a posttransfusion blood specimen, submitting the remaining blood with tag and tubing to the blood bank, sending the first posttransfusion urine specimen to the laboratory for analysis of free hemoglobin, and symptomatically and supportively treating the patient.

Analysis of blood and urine samples may give an indication as to the cause of the reaction and aid the physician in determining appropriate follow-up therapy.

DISSEMINATED INTRAVASCULAR COAGULATION (DIC)

Disseminated intravascular coagulation (DIC) is classified as the oldest universally accepted hypercoagulable state known. Synonyms for DIC are consumption coagulopathy, diffuse intravascular clotting, and defibrination syndrome.

In order that an understanding of DIC be meaningful, an understanding of the in vitro and in vivo mechanisms of clotting is necessary.

The in vitro mechanism of clotting is as follows: because of enzymatic action that alters the clotting factors, blood will clot when it is removed from the body and placed in or on an untreated surface. Clots form when factor XII is activated and converted into an enzyme. This enzyme then converts factor XI to an enzyme. Factor VIII activates factor X and factor V activates prothrombin. The platelet cofactor-3 must be present to activate both factors VIII and V. A self-perpetuating effect as described by Hudak et al. (1973) takes place by activating factor X through the effect of thrombin on factor VIII. A fibrin clot forms when thrombin converts fibrinogen.

The body's natural antagonist to this process is the fibrinolytic system. Several proenzymes within this system serve to dissolve clots. The dissolving enzyme is called plasmin. The state of this system can be determined by assessing plasmin blood levels.

The in vivo mechanism activates only when repair of blood vessels is needed. Any tear in the epithelial lining of a blood vessel will attract platelets. With platelet buildup at the site of a tear, normal blood flow and current is altered. This activates the clotting mechanism and can actually cause further platelet buildup, since thrombin is released and an eventual occlusion of the vessel may ensue. However, the fibrinolytic system keeps a balance between clot formation and clot lysis (Hudak et al., 1973). The balance is disturbed when there is an imbalance of the necessary factors such as decreased factor VIII as in hemophilia and increased or decreased fibrinolytic factors.

DIC is a syndrome that occurs secondary to several diseases. The coagulability of blood is altered, resulting in an increased tendency to clot.

Patients who develop DIC are usually in a state of hypotension and shock with vasoconstriction and capillary dilation. Blood bypasses the capillaries and therefore capillary circulation is poor. The capillary blood becomes acidotic after a short time. Certain coagulation substances present in the blood, such as free hemoglobin, toxins, placental tissue, amniotic fluid, and cancer tissue fragments may precipitate DIC. It may also be precipitated during open heart surgery when the extracorporeal pump is inadequately prepared.

The process of DIC is rapid. Most of the clotting factors are soon used up and hemostasis is lost. This results in bleeding. Stress activates the fibrinolytic system, causing an increase in fibrinolysis, which enhances bleeding.

An excessive amount of thrombin forms and converts fibrinogen to fibrin clots. Transfusions of blood, fibrinogen, and plasma serve only to continue the syndrome and hemorrhage. All naturally occurring antithrombins are usually absent.

Treatment of DIC involves removing the cause and controlling the clotting-hemorrhage cycle through the administration of heparin. Heparin neutralizes thrombin and acts as an anticoagulant. Heparin administered for this purpose must be administered intravenously in order to assure absorption of the medication, to prevent local hematoma, and to provide for immediate effect. The usual dosage is 10,000 to 20,000 units every 2 to 4 hours. IV push is the preferred method. The actual dosage is determined by therapeutic blood levels of heparin. Acid-base balance must be restored.

Once the clotting factors are restored through natural methods, the heparin is gradually discontinued.

References

Abbott Laboratories: The use of blood, North Chicago, Ill., 1966, Abbott Laboratories.

Alton Ochsner Medical Foundation, Hospital Division, Departments of Nursing and Blood Bank: Policy and procedure manual, New Orleans, 1977, The Foundation.

American Association of Blood Banks: Blood component therapy—a physician's handbook, Washington, D.C., 1975, The Association.

Beland, I., and Passos, J.: Textbook of medical-surgical nursing, ed. 3, Philadelphia, 1975, J. B. Lippincott Co.

Brunner, L., and Suddarth, D.: Textbook of medical-surgical nursing, ed. 3, Philadelphia, 1975, J. B. Lippincott Co.

Flexner, J.: Uses and abuses of blood, Intravenous therapy in-service training series clinical seminar no. 1, 1967.

Hudak, C., et al.: Critical care nursing, In Altschuler, J.: Disseminated intravascular coagulation syndrome, Philadelphia, 1973, J. B. Lippincott Co.

Plumer, A.: Principles and practice of intravenous therapy, ed. 2, Boston, 1975, Little, Brown & Co.

Rossman, M., Slavin, R., and Taft, E. G.: Pheresis therapy: patient care, Am. J. Nurs. **77:**7, July 1977.

Thomas, C., editor: Taber's cyclopedic medical dictionary, ed. 13, Philadelphia, 1977, F. A. Davis Co.

Snively, W., and Beshear, D.: Textbook of pathophysiology, Philadelphia, 1972, J. B. Lippincott Co.

U.S. Department of Health, Education, and Welfare, Public Health Service: Food and Drug Administration Drug Bull. **8:**5, Oct.-Nov. 1978.

Appendix A

Formulas for calculating drug dosages

$$\frac{\text{Dose desired}}{\text{Dose on hand}} \times \text{Volume} \left(\frac{D}{H} \times V \right)$$

Example: The physician orders diazepam, 2.5 mg, to be administered. On hand is 10 mg in 2 ml. How many milliliters are to be administered?

$$\frac{2.5 \text{ mg}}{10 \text{ mg}} \times 2 \text{ ml} = 0.5 \text{ ml}$$

Example: The physician orders atropine gr $^1\!/_{75}$ to be administered. On hand is gr $^1\!/_{150}$ in 1 ml. How many ml are to be administered?

$$\frac{\text{gr } ^1\!/_{75}}{\text{gr } ^1\!/_{150}} \times 1 = \frac{1}{75} \times \frac{150}{1} = \frac{150}{75} = 2 \text{ ml}$$

Appendix B

Formulas for calculating IV flow rates in ml/hour, drops/hour, drops/minute, and ml/minute

ML/HOUR

$$\frac{\text{Total ml fluid to be given}}{\text{Total hours to be administered}} = \text{ml/hour}$$

Example: $\dfrac{1000 \text{ ml}}{8 \text{ hrs}} = 125 \text{ ml/hour}$

DROPS/HOUR

$$\text{Desired ml/hour} \times \text{Drops/ml} = \text{Drops/hour}$$

Example: 125 ml × 10 = 1250 drops/hour. Drops/ml is determined by tubing drop factor.

DROPS/MINUTE

$$\frac{\text{Desired drops/hour}}{60 \text{ minutes}} = \text{Drops/minute}$$

Example: $\dfrac{1250 \text{ drops}}{60 \text{ minutes}} = 20.8$ or 21 drops/minute

ML/MINUTE

$$\frac{\text{ml/hour}}{60 \text{ minutes}} \times \frac{x}{1 \text{ minute}}$$

Example: $60x = 125$
$x = 20.8$ or 21 ml/minute

Tubing drop factors range from 10, 15, and 60 drops/ml.

Since microdrop sets have 60 drops/ml, the rule is that drops/minute will represent ml/hour. That is to say, should 125 ml be required in 1 hour, the rate of flow will be 125 drops/minute; 50 ml/hour, 50 drops/minute, and so on.

157

Bibliography

American Medical Association: AMA drug evaluations, ed. 3, Prepared by American Medical Association Department of Drugs in cooperation with the American Society for Clinical Pharmacology and Therapeutics, Littleton, Mass., 1977, Publishing Science Group, Inc.

Cooper, S.: Drug administration and the law, RN, Jan. 1961.

Edwards, L., and Barker, K.: Pharmacology notes for nurses, Am. J. Nurs. **62**:10, Oct. 1962.

Hayt, E., et al.: Law of hospital and nurse, New York, 1958, Hospital Textbook Co.

Henderson, V., and Nite, G.: Principles and practice of nursing, ed. 6, New York, 1978, The Macmillan Co.

Hussar, D.: Cardiac drugs today—anticoagulants, Nursing 73, April 1973.

Imperiale, M., and Virebs, T.: The intravenous therapy nurses, Am. J. Nurs. **61**:5, May 1961.

Johns, M.: Pharmacodynamics and patient care, St. Louis, 1974, The C. V. Mosby Co.

Johnson, N.: Coping with complications of intravenous therapy, Nursing 72, Feb. 1972.

Kron, T.: Stepping beyong the five rights of administering drugs, Am. J. Nurs. **62**:7, July 1962.

Maki, D., et al.: Infection control in intravenous therapy, Nurs. Digest, May-June 1975.

Manzi, C., and Masoorli, S.: Trouble with IV's, Nursing 78, Oct. 1978.

Miller, B., and Keane, C.: Encyclopedia and dictionary of medicine and nursing, Philadelphia, 1972, W. B. Saunders Co.

Molyneau-Luici, M.: The ABCs of multiple trauma, Nursing 77 **7**:10, Oct. 1977.

Moore, V.: IV fluids, Nursing 73, June 1973.

Payne, J., and Kaplan, H.: Alternative techniques for venipuncture, Am. J. Nurs. **72**:4, April 1972.

Rodman, M., and Smith, D.: Clinical pharmacology in nursing, Philadelphia, 1974, J. B. Lippincott Co.

St. Joseph Hospital Medical Center, Burbank, Calif.: Nursing service procedure manual, St. Louis, 1971, The Catholic Hospital Association.

Scranton, P.: Practical techniques in venipuncture, Baltimore, 1977, The Williams & Wilkins Co.

Chapter 1

Alsobrook, H.: Liability prevention, Institutional and personal seminar, New Orleans, 1976.

Creighton, H.: Law every nurse should know, ed. 2, Philadelphia, 1970, W. B. Saunders Co.

Lesnik, M., and Anderson, B.: Nursing practice and the law, ed. 2, Philadelphia, 1962, J. B. Lippincott Co.

Chapter 2

Borris, G., et al.: Inflammatory potential of foreign particulates, Anesth. Analg. **56**:3, May-June 1977.

Center for Disease Control: Recommendations for the prevention of IV-associated infections, Atlanta, 1973, Bacterial Diseases Branch, Bureau of Epidemiology.

Concept media: Infection control and IV therapy, selected readings, Costa Mesa, Calif., 1973, Concept Media.

Francke, D.: Handbook of IV additive review, Drug intelligence publication, Hamilton, Ill., 1973, The Hamilton Press.

Goldmann, D. A., Maki, D. G., Rhame, F. S., et al.: Guidelines for infection control in intravenous therapy, Ann. Intern. Med. **79**:848, Dec. 1973.

Goldmann, D. A., Martin, W. T., and Worthington, J. W.: Growth of bacteria and fungi in total parenteral nutrition solutions, Am. J. Surg., **126**:314, Sept. 1973.

Isler, C.: IV therapy: the hidden dangers, RN vol. 10, Oct. 1973.

Maki, D. G., Goldmann, D. A., and Rhame, F. S.: Infection control in intravenous therapy, Ann. Intern. Med. **79**:867, Dec. 1973.

Plumer, A.: Principles and practice of intravenous therapy, ed. 2, Boston, 1975, Little, Brown & Co.

Rebagay, T., Rapp, R., Bivins, B., et al.: Residues in antibiotic preparations: scanning electron microscopic studies of surface topography, Am. J. Hosp. Pharm. **33**:433, May 1976.

Rusmin, S., Althauser, M. B., and DeLuca, P. P.: Consequences of microbial contamination during extended intravenous therapy using in-line filters, Am. J. Hosp. Pharm., **32**:373, April 1975.

Chapter 3

Abbott Laboratories: Venipuncture and venous cannulation, North Chicago, Ill., Aug. 1972, Abbott Laboratories.

Brunner, L., and Suddarth, D.: Textbook of medical-surgical nursing, ed. 3, Philadelphia, 1975, J. B. Lippincott Co.

Goss, C., editor: Gray's anatomy, ed. 27, Philadelphia, 1959, Lea & Febiger.

Guyton, A.: Functions of the human body, ed. 4, Philadelphia, 1974, W. B. Saunders Co.

Johnson, W. H., et al.: Biology, ed. 4, New York, 1972, Holt, Rinehart & Winston.

Chapter 4

Endicott, C.: Workshop on parenteral incompatibilities, Am. J. Hosp. Pharm. **23**:599, 1966.

Johnson, W. H., et al.: Biology, ed. 4, New York, 1972, Holt, Rinehart & Winston.

Kabat, H.: Intravenous incompatibility, Abbott Laboratories, Health care worldwide, Intravenous therapy in-service training series, clinical seminar no. 2, 1971.

Keenan, C., and Wood, J.: General college chemistry, ed. 4, New York, 1971, Harper & Row, Publishers.

Musser, R., and O'Neill, J.: Pharmacology and therapeutics, ed. 4, New York, 1969, Macmillan Publishing Co.

Chapter 5

Abbott Laboratories: Fluid and electrolytes, North Chicago, Ill., 1969, Abbott Laboratories.

Anthony, C.: Fluid imbalances—formidable foes to survival, Am. J. Nurs. **63**:12, Dec. 1963.

Beland, I., and Passos, J.: Clinical nursing, ed. 3, New York, 1975, Macmillan Publishing Co.

Burns, W., and Crawford, D.: Indications for intravenous therapy and the nurse's responsibility, Abbott Laboratories, Intravenous therapy in-service training series, clinical seminar no. 4, 1971.

Kee, J.: The critically ill patient and possible fluid and electrolyte imbalances, Nursing 72, March 1972.

Methany, N., and Snively, W.: Nurses' handbook of fluid balance, Philadelphia, 1967, J. B. Lippincott Co.

Moore, V. B.: IV fluids, Nursing 73, June 1973.

Chapter 6

Beland, I., and Passos, J.: Clinical nursing, ed. 3, New York, 1975, Macmillan Publishing Co.

Johnson, W. H., et al.: Biology, ed. 4, New York, 1972, Holt, Rinehart & Winston.

Chapter 7

Alton Ochsner Medical Foundation, Hospital Division, Pharmacy Department, New Orleans, 1977.

Brunner, L., and Suddarth, D.: Textbook of medical-surgical nursing, ed. 3, Philadelphia, 1975, J. B. Lippincott Co.

Dudrick, S., and Rhoads, J.: Total intravenous feeding, Sci. Am. **226**:73, 1972.

Johnson, C., et al.: Parenteral hyperalimentation, Lexington, Ky., 1973, University of Kentucky College of Pharmacy.

Johnson, W. H., et al.: Biology, ed. 4, New York, 1972, Holt, Rinehart & Winston.

Kaminski, M.: Total parenteral nutrition (hyperalimentation): prevention and treatment of complications, a policy and procedure manual, Registery, Washington, D.C., Nov. 1972, Walter Reed General Hospital.

Plumer, A.: Principles and practice of intravenous therapy, ed. 2, Boston, 1975, Little, Brown & Co.

Purdue Frederick Co.: Recommendations for

infection control during IV hyperalimentation, Norwalk, Conn., 1974, Purdue Frederick Co.

Rapp, M., et al.: Hyperalimentation, RN, Aug. 1976.

Upjohn Laboratories: Parenteral hyperalimentation, Kalamazoo, Mich., June 1971, The Upjohn Co.

Chapter 8

Barbier, S.: Blood can't be bought but its price tag is high, Times Picayune Newspaper (New Orleans), sect. 2, page 2, April 24, 1978.

Gahart, B.: Intravenous medications—a handbook for nurses and other allied health personnel, ed. 2, St. Louis, 1977, The C. V. Mosby Co.

Jensen, M. D., Benson, R. C., and Bobak, I. M.: Maternity care, St. Louis, 1977, The C. V. Mosby Co.

Johnson, W. H., et al.: Biology, ed. 4, New York, 1972, Holt, Rinehart, & Winston.

Methany, N., and Snively, W.: Nurses' handbook of fluid balance, Philadelphia, 1967, J. B. Lippincott Co.

O'Brien, B., and Woods, S.: The paradox of DIC, Am. J. Nurs. **78**:11, Nov. 1978.

Tenczynski, J.: Leukapheresis—the process, Am. J. Nurs. **77**:7, July 1977.

Index